The Big Book of Tai Chi

Other books by Bruce Frantzis

The Power of Internal Martial Arts
Opening the Energy Gates of Your Body
Relaxing into Your Being
The Great Stillness

The Big Book of Tai Chi

BUILD HEALTH FAST IN SLOW MOTION

BRUCE FRANTZIS

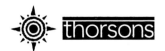
thorsons

Thorsons
An Imprint of HarperCollins*Publishers*
77–85 Fulham Palace Road
Hammersmith, London W6 8JB

The Thorsons website is www.thorsonselement.com

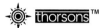

and Thorsons are registered trade marks
of HarperCollins*Publishers* Ltd

First published in 2003

1 3 5 7 9 10 8 6 4 2

© Bruce Frantzis, 2003

Bruce Frantzis asserts the moral right to
be identified as the author of this work

A catalogue record for this book
is available from the British Library

ISBN 0 00 713090 2

Printed and bound in Great Britain by
Scotprint, Haddington, East Lothian

Front cover photograph by Michael McKee,
with models Faye Baker, Dorothy Fitzer, and Alistair Shanks

Studio photography by Guy Hearn

PLEASE NOTE: While the author of this book has made every effort to ensure that the information
contained in this book is as accurate and up-to-date as possible at the time of publication, medical and
pharmaceutical knowledge is constantly changing and the application of it to particular circumstances
depends on many factors. This book should not be used as an alternative to specialist medical advice and it
is recommended that readers always consult a qualified medical professional for individual advice before
following any new diet or health programme. The author and publishers cannot be held responsible for any
errors and omissions that may be found in the text, or any actions that may be taken by a reader, as a result
of any reliance on the information contained in the text, which are taken entirely at the reader's own risk.

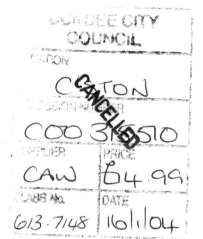

Contents

Chapter 4: How Tai Chi Reduces and Manages Stress 65

This book is dedicated to all the people in the future who will benefit from tai chi, whatever tradition they learn.

Author's Note

My purpose is to share ideas about how and why tai chi works to stimulate thought and further inquiry. My experience of studying in China for 11 years with masters in tai chi and chi gung has given me a unique perspective. I hope this book will encourage scientists to make formal studies of tai chi's health benefits, inspire people to try tai chi, and provide tools to enable current tai chi practitioners and instructors to upgrade their skills and gain more benefit and satisfaction from their practice.

Acknowledgements

My profound thanks to all my teachers without whom it would have been impossible to write this book. I owe especial gratitude to the late Liu Hung Chieh, who, in the last years of his life, put so much of his effort into training me so that I could spread the benefits of tai chi to the West.

I wish to acknowledge all the tai chi teachers who are working hard to bring this valuable art to people all over the world in the hope of benefiting the human condition.

My gratitude goes to many. First to all my students and the instructors I have trained, whose genuine interest was the motivation for writing this book and who have shared their invaluable insights on how to make this book particularly relevant to modern life.

Many reviewed drafts of the manuscript and gave suggestions that helped make this a better book. In particular, Bill Ryan, founder of Brookline Tai Chi in Boston, Massachusetts, who has trained with me for twenty years, gave me many valuable comments. He paid careful and patient attention to detail while reviewing all the many versions of the manuscript.

I also want to give special thanks to my friend Diane Rapaport, whom I have trained as an instructor, for the time she generously spent throughout this entire project. Her editing helped make this book clearer and better organized.

Thank you to the following for reviewing and providing medical information: Melinda

Franceschini, who is pursuing a Ph.D. in Stress Physiology in the Department of Biology at Tufts University, Massachuetts; Marie-Helene Jouvin, M.D., Research Associate, Harvard Medical School; and John and Angela Hicks, founders of The College of Integrated Chinese Medicine, Reading, UK, one of the UK's most prominent acupuncture schools. Angela Hicks is also the author of *The Five Secrets of Health and Happiness*.

Thank you to Alan Peatfield, Ph.D., College Lecturer in Greek Archeology at University College Dublin, for reviewing some of Taoism's historical traditions.

I'm also grateful to Wanda Whiteley, Acquisitions Editor at Thorsons, for her vision in seeing the value of this book, to her colleague Susanna Abbot, for shepherding the book through its many editorial phases, and to Charlotte Ridings, for careful final editing.

I wish to thank all the photographers and models who contributed pictures to this book, especially Guy Hearn, photographer for the UK shoot, with models Megan Fisher, Cleophas Gaillard, Hoa Luc, Sarah Majid, and Vicky Maschio; and Michael McKee, photographer for the USA shoot, with models Faye Baker, Dorothy Fitzer, Pat Krock, Angel Negrete and Alistair Shanks.

A special thank you to the staff at Energy Arts: Art Director, Michael McKee for creating the book's illustrations and for his photographic and design assistance; Hyacin Rosser-Wolff, Chief of Operations; Cathy Bleecker, Events Manager; and Martha McKee, Office Manager, for handling some of the minutiae and communications that are so integral to a book's creation. Thanks also to graphic designer Faye Baker, whom I trained as a tai chi instructor, for helping to organize photographs and illustrations for this book.

Finally, thanks to my wife Caroline, former BBC journalist, for all her love, support, and humor. She kept the chaos in our lives to a manageable din so I could have more time to write. A better writer than I, she has significantly improved this book with her superb copyediting skills and photo research.

Foreword

Getting Older; Feeling Younger

by Diane Rapaport

Bruce Frantzis' life story could be the basis of a Hollywood movie. When he was 18, he turned down a scholarship at Harvard, sold his possessions, and left Manhattan to spend 15 of the next 20 years in Japan, India, and China to devote himself to training in the 3,000-year-old Eastern tradition of warrior, healer, and priest. He already held black belts in karate, aikido, judo, and jujitsu.

Frantzis trained in arts whose secrets had been kept inaccessible to Westerners and coped with old and embedded Oriental prejudices. He became fluent in Japanese and Chinese and earned great distinction and respect. He trained with championship judo and karate teams in Tokyo, Japan; earned an acupuncture degree in Hong Kong; worked as a chi gung therapist in cancer wards in Chinese hospitals; trained with the most highly regarded martial artists; and earned three of the highest positions in the Taoist hierarchy: Master of the Taoist Arts, Formal Disciple, and Lineage Holder. In China, these titles are given only to someone exceptionally skilled at the highest levels of Taoist martial arts, which include tai chi, *ba gua*, and *hsing-i*, as well as other energy arts, including chi gung and meditation.

The only higher positions are that of Head of a Lineage and Chinese Immortal. Both of these were titles held by Liu Hung Chieh, Bruce's most eminent teacher.

Liu said of Bruce: "When I tell him 'A' he already knows 'Z.' He understands everything from his heart and soul. He is diligent and practices hard. He is very humble when he asks questions. In one day of practice he can go a thousand miles. I am very happy that he is a very special and outstanding student."

First Encounters

For many, Bruce's background as a healer, warrior, and priest might conjure up images of the venerable, soft-spoken man that was David Carradine's teacher in the *Kung Fu* television series, or the lean, handsome bearing of Chow Yun Fat, star of the film *Crouching Tiger, Hidden Dragon*. But these images in no way prepared me for the reality of meeting Bruce Frantzis for the first time and attending his classes.

My first encounter with Bruce was through my husband Walt, who had been diagnosed with emphysema. My daughter insisted that he spend an hour talking with Bruce. I was skeptical. What could anyone do in an hour?

Walt described his meeting this way: "I saw this huge guy come lumbering into the room, swaying from side to side. As he ambled closer and closer, his first words to me were, 'What's wrong with you?' As soon as I got the word 'emphysema' out of my mouth, Bruce engulfed me in his arms. He asked me to breathe. I didn't have time to put up any defenses, so I just did it."

Bruce told Walt that he was a shallow breather who had only used a small portion of his lungs for a long time, which caused healthy portions of the lung to atrophy. "Bruce showed me how it was possible to breathe into different parts of my lungs—lower side right, upper back, left, etc. He explained that by learning to reactivate unused portions of my lungs I could restore functionality and compensate for the damage that had occurred."

Walt came home a different man. He had lost much of his fearfulness about his illness, and, though his breath was still shallow, it was not labored and ponderous. "Bruce taught me some very practical skills to take control of my health problems and do something for myself."

This was a very different approach from that of the doctors and alternative healers we had encountered. None had suggested that we could heal ourselves directly, nor taught the skills that could do so. Instead, they told us that they could heal us with their skills and whatever combination of drugs and vitamins they sold. Later, I learned that the Taoist definition of a mature human being is someone who takes responsibility for him- or herself and does not blame someone else for their miseries, and, if possible, does not continually seek out someone that will cure them of whatever ails them.

I was intrigued. I let go of my skepticism and decided to check this man out.

The first time I met Bruce was at a Thanksgiving party. Even though Walt had described him as "huge" I was not really prepared for someone that looked like a bear. He combined the intellectual breadth of a Renaissance scholar with the laid back guilelessness of a child. He spoke and ate with gargantuan gusto. But it was his dancing to the music of The Jefferson Airplane that destroyed my preconceived notions about what warriors, healers, and priests might be like, and gave me some insight into less obvious powers. The bear disappeared and Bruce turned into a butterfly. He had a lightness, speed, and unselfconscious grace that did not at all fit with his ambling shuffle and size. He changed direction effortlessly with relaxed agility. As though sensing my astonishment, he suddenly turned to me and with an ingenuous grin said, "I was responsible for starting a tai chi disco craze in China."

First Class Encounters: Relaxation

I signed up for one of Bruce's week-long tai chi summer retreats in California, which started three weeks after my 55th birthday. I was recovering from the effects of a bronchial infection that had kicked my allergies and asthma into high gear and had left me feeling stressed and depleted. It was my third bronchial illness that year and I had been taking strong antibiotics, using inhalers twice daily to restrain the asthma, and using antihistamines for the allergies. I had virtually no sense of smell or taste. I had bursitis in my left shoulder and arthritis in my finger joints. Old age seemed to be coming on fast and I was quite motivated to learn something that would help me feel better.

After Bruce walked into class, he looked for a few moments at the 90 students, who had come from a great variety of countries. "Now," he announced with no fanfare, "one fundamental principle of tai chi is to relax the mind and body; and the way tai chi accomplishes this is to train you to use energy, not muscles, to move your body. Stretch out your arms," he said. "put them as far out ahead of you as you can. Stretch. Stretch more. And hold your arms in that position for a few moments." When he asked us to drop our arms, there was a unanimous sigh of relief. "Tensing the muscles tenses the mind and the body and tires you out. It decreases circulation, especially to the internal organs. That's why stress is killing us. Ever hear of anyone going to the hospital for a relaxation attack?"

Then Bruce introduced an exercise that showed us how easy it was to stretch our arms out even farther when they were relaxed and empty of tension. In this simple and direct way, Bruce immediately focused our attention directly on our bodies. His goal was to get us out of our heads into the reality of what we were doing and feeling. "From the outside in," is an old adage of the ancient Chinese book of wisdom, the *Tao Te Ching*. It is one of the fundamental underpinnings of tai chi. The body is the point of entry that takes us deeper and deeper into our minds and spirit.

Like many people, I had ignored my body. It was just a piece of battered luggage that I carted around. I did not like to look at myself. I did not feel the distinct parts of my body, much less my internal organs and nervous system. I had never tried. I did not think it was important. And it was a long time into my tai chi practice before I came to understand the deep connections between places that were tense in my body and emotional blockages and disease.

Alignments

All my life, well-meaning parents and teachers told me to stand up straight. But no one ever taught me what standing up straight meant. Did it mean tucking in the belly, or thrusting the chest out? Did it mean locking the joints of the knees and hips? By the time that I was 55, I had very poor posture. I had pigeon-toed feet and walked with a stooped, forward thrust that had arched my back into a light scoliosis. My friends called it my "chicken walk." The posture locked up my shoulders and neck so that headaches were commonplace.

In his classes, Bruce systematically taught the components of good posture, joint by joint, and showed how to apply them to each movement of tai chi. He would demonstrate a particular movement and then in precise, clear detail break it down into all its components: how to hold the wrist and elbow; how to keep the shoulders from rising; how to correctly bend at the hip; how to shift the weight from the back foot to the front foot. In one class, we studied the proper alignment of the ankle joint, and learned how collapsed arches could be slowly corrected; another was on the correct alignment of the hip, knee, and ankle joints so that no weight and strain would be put on the knee.

Bruce taught many supplementary exercises and gave demonstrations that boggled credulity. In one, he asked a petite young woman to lie flat on her back with one leg in the air. He put his hand on the bottom of her foot, manipulated her leg from the hip in a variety of positions, and asked her to move his hand. In incorrect positions, she would feel a twinge in her knee when she pressed against his hand and she could not move it. With the correct alignment, she could easily use her leg to shift any pressure he applied.

Once she felt where the correct alignment was, Bruce asked the largest man in the class to put his full weight on the bottom of her foot. She easily pumped him back and forth with absolutely no strain on her knee. Then he asked a second man to lean on the first. She easily moved two people. By the time she had six men putting their full weight on the bottom of her foot and was moving all of them back and forth, we were totally amazed.

"Are you using any tension to move them?" Bruce asked.

"No."

"Is there any pain?"

"None."

"Is it difficult?"

"Hardly at all," she said with a big grin on her face.

Teaching Style

Bruce's classes are 80 percent physical and 20 percent theory and philosophy. His is a down-to-earth teaching style with a lot of hands-on work among the students. Nothing is made to seem esoteric, unusual, inaccessible, secretive, or mysterious, including the flow of energy, or chi. He did not try to motivate us with pep talks. He did not approve or disapprove when moves were done poorly or well. He showed no favoritism or bias toward any students, even those who were the most gifted.

"Everyone has different aptitudes and learns at different speeds," Bruce said. "You are not in competition with anyone in this class. Thinking about how you look and comparing yourself with others sets you up for frustration and emotional pain. Tai chi isn't something that you can learn by watching or thinking about it; true transformation is only attained with effort. If you practice, your body will lose tension and gain health, stamina, and vitality."

This is not to say that Bruce taught everyone the same way. His classes were filled with students who were working at different levels of practice. There were people that were learning the physical movements—the basic alphabet of tai chi; intermediate students learning how to feel and relax deeper layers inside their bodies; and advanced students who were discovering the subtleties of how energy could be directed in the body for healing, self-defense, or meditation.

Bruce has a remarkable gift for being able to hone in on what each student needs to advance to the next stage of their practice, and makes sure that he gives them that missing piece. Sometimes he would make a very slight adjustment of a student's head or gently twist their arm to release tension. Sometimes he would demonstrate a self-defense maneuver to help students remember a move or make an energy transmission to help them understand what to feel inside their bodies.

I did not know how unusual Bruce's teaching style was because I had nothing to compare it with. But during the last seven years, I have heard many of Bruce's students say, "I learned more in one class here than I did in the past twenty years." Certainly, few Westerners have the comprehensive knowledge of tai chi that is needed to explain its complexities, and many Chinese practitioners don't have the language to make what they know comprehensible, and are reluctant to impart what they consider secret knowledge. Bruce shares his knowledge openly, contravening the normal practice of withholding secrets except to a chosen few. His teacher Liu understood that the days of needing to protect martial arts secrets were over and that those same secrets could greatly benefit the health of millions.

Bruce's gift is that he has the expert knowledge and intelligence to translate the Chinese concepts into English and bridge the East-West gap, making this subject comprehensible to everyone.

Feeling Younger; Getting Older

Tai chi is low-impact exercise done in slow motion. Its effects are as gradual, natural, and inexorable as water etching out a canyon. Tai chi's gentleness and lack of pain and strain mean that everyone can do it and gain benefits. In Bruce's words, "Even the poorest quality tai chi practice, done steadfastly, will nourish the body and mind and give you one of the most inexpensive and satisfying meals you'll ever encounter."

Because so much of my focus during the first year of practice was taken up with remembering—and being frustrated at forgetting—the moves and basic alignments and weight shifts, I did not notice a major change in my health right away. But one night as I prepared for sleep I realized that I was not putting on woolen socks to keep my feet warm. Then I remembered that I hadn't been putting on any socks for weeks and that my feet were seldom cold anymore. "Right," I thought, "tai chi improves circulation."

The second marker was when I noticed that I had developed enough body consciousness to tune into a headache coming on, and relax the muscles around my head and in the back of the center of the eyes to stop it. Bruce would say in class, "Tai chi makes the body conscious." I did not know what that meant when I first heard it.

The third was an emotional breakthrough. I understood that the weakness in my lungs was due to some deeply embedded constrictions that were slowly choking me to death. During my month-long tai chi instructor training, a great deal of energy got turned loose. It was as though a roller-coaster was free inside my body and I could not guard against its steep pitches. Grief and sadness were dominant and I could not push them back with my usual defenses. Early memories of being forced to eat foods I did not like, my father's anger when I gulped too loudly at dinner, and the deeper grief at my father's abandonment of my mother led me to adopt the defense mechanisms of locking my throat against taste, constricting my lungs instead of crying, and using my allergies to get sympathy.

Over time, I layered those mechanisms with what I thought were more positive ones—charm, intellect, and skill at helping others solve business and aesthetic challenges. But all of these were methods to shelter my emotions and lock people out. I wanted approval for my good deeds and I did not want others to see my emotional weaknesses. I kept myself hidden—not only from others, but from myself. With these discoveries came the tears that I had held back for many years, which I let run until they were truly spent. Then began the much harder work of focusing on my weaknesses, not my strengths, and releasing tensions that remained in my body, which were the remnants of those ill-conceived defenses.

When I told Bruce what had happened, he simply said with a wry smile, "Denial is not just a river in Egypt."

At 63, I am a different person than I was at 55. I haven't had bronchitis for three winters now. My allergies have all but disappeared. I can go for months at a time without using inhalers. I no longer have that stooped chicken walk. And I have the energy and stamina I had in my early thirties. I can work seven hours at my computer, come home, do a few tai chi sets, lose the day's tensions and feel energized. I can go river rafting, and row five or six miles without feeling totally wasted at the end of the day.

The effect on my mind and spirit is equally dramatic. I feel a new approach to life opening up, one based on freedom from competition, approval, and aggression. I have an easier, less judgmental approach to myself and to others. Most astonishing, the more relaxed I feel, the more clarity and energy I have. So many of the conditionings of upbringing and society are slowly peeling away as I practice these graceful, slow-motion movements. I am drawn deeper and deeper into self-exploration and discovery, and feel my spirit and heart opening up.

Yes, I'm getting older, but I'm feeling younger.

Tai Chi and the Health Crisis

Bruce Frantzis teaches tai chi to help people achieve health, relaxation, and longevity. He is a teacher with a mission:

> Tai chi is the one exercise that can universally help solve our growing health crisis. It has stood the test of thousands of years. We have a generation of baby boomers with increasing health problems; old people who are sick, in pain, fearful, and cranky; a middle class that is increasingly becoming incapable of affording most of the drugs that are prescribed for their ailments; children that are flaccid, diabetic, and asthmatic. People of all ages are addicted to drugs, alcohol, sugar, cigarettes, and caffeine. Stress follows almost everyone like a shadow.
>
> But at the very base of this health crisis is the cancerous spiritual malaise in the West, a fundamental disharmony that keeps people from positively engaging with life and relaxing in virtually any circumstances that life can throw.
>
> Tai chi is about changing our internal environment so that life becomes a joy to live and not a burden to drag into old age and death. It is about helping your body to let go of the past and your mind to slow down and cease churning. Tai chi encourages your internal focus to shift toward cherishing and remembering all that is wonderful in your life. It predisposes you to look forward to ways to make life better, rather than remembering how unsatisfying it has been.
>
> Most importantly, tai chi gives us the ability to realize a greater human potential in ourselves and to have genuine compassion for others. Tai chi, with its gentle strength, moves us closer to feeling more truly alive.

This seminal book explains in detail how and why tai chi can help you experience full aliveness in your physical, emotional, intellectual, and spiritual life.

Is there anyone that doesn't need to feel more alive?

Diane Rapaport is the author of *How To Make and Sell Your Own Recording* and *A Music Business Primer*, published by Prentice Hall. She has been studying with Bruce Frantzis since 1995 and has been trained by him as a tai chi and chi gung instructor.

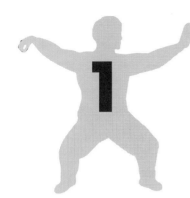

What is Tai Chi?

We recognize tai chi when we see people doing a series of silent, fluid, seamless slow-motion movements. Because it looks so peaceful and relaxed, many assume that the participants are involved in some form of meditation. Some may notice that these graceful movements resemble kicks, punches, and chops.

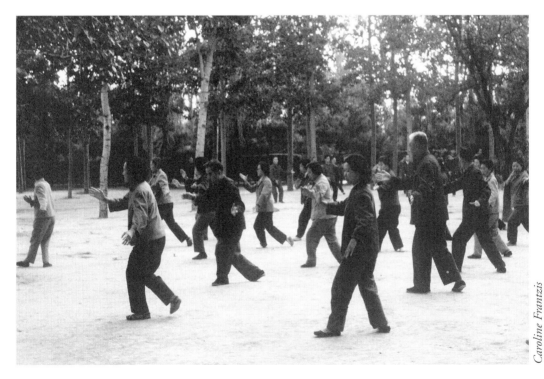

Caroline Frantzis

Tai chi is practiced by millions of people every morning in public parks throughout China

This is because tai chi was developed in China as a very effective martial art. Distinct styles were developed within specific families as a means of protection and were named after their founders: Wu, Chen, Yang, Hao, etc. Each style has a series of distinct choreographed movements called forms, with short ones lasting only for a few minutes and the longest ones up to an hour. Each style has many variations.

Today, millions of people in the Western world practice tai chi to gain its practical benefits: reduced stress, improved health and longevity, and lifelong vitality and stamina.

In China, tai chi is the national health exercise. Over 200 million people practice tai chi daily, more than any other martial art in the world. Everyone has a relative, friend, or co-worker who regularly does tai chi. Everyone knows it is really good for health; no one has to tell them. While living in Taiwan during my twenties, I often encountered older Chinese people who politely asked what I was doing in China. When I told them I was practicing tai chi, there was usually a concerned look as they solemnly asked in broken English, "What kind of sick have you got?"

However, as most Chinese martial artists know, the tiny percentage of people that practice tai chi for self-defense are not to be taken lightly. Nevertheless, you do not have to be a martial arts master to gain tai chi's benefits. Nor do you have to be classically fit, athletic, or intelligent. Unlike many exercise systems or sports, one valuable aspect of tai chi is that it can be done by anyone who can stand up; and it has specific adaptations for people confined to wheelchairs. You can do tai chi if you are fat or thin, healthy or just out of bed after major surgery, young, middle-aged, or very old.

In China, half of all participants take up tai chi between the ages of 50 and 80, or even older, when the need to overcome the potential negative effects of aging cannot be denied. Others practice to enhance their physical and intellectual capabilities. Competition athletes use tai chi to improve their reflexes and reduce the time it takes to heal from sports injuries. Tai chi helps middle-aged people to cope with the ever-increasing responsibilities of life, reduce stress, and get a competitive edge in business. Still others use tai chi to develop inner discipline, open their heart and mind, and unleash their spiritual potential.

Like anything that has really stood the test of time, there is a lot more to tai chi than first impressions. Tai chi contains important parts of the accumulated wisdom of the ancient world, and can help everyone overcome the ever-present difficulties of the human condition and engage with life positively.

The Meaning of *Tai Chi Chuan*

Tai chi chuan is the full name of what many people simply refer to as "tai chi." It is composed of two separate ideas. The first, *tai chi*, encompasses philosophical and spiritual concepts; the second, *chuan*, which literally means fist or boxing, encompasses its martial arts or warrior aspects.

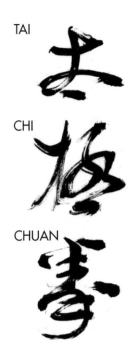

TAI

CHI

CHUAN

The Meaning of *Tai Chi*

Tai (pronounced like the tie in bow *tie*) literally means large or great. The word *chi* (pronounced like the gee of *gee* whiz) connotes the superlative of a word, such as biggest, richest, deepest. So *tai chi* literally means "the maximum biggest," and is often translated by variations on the same theme such as "the supreme ultimate," "the grand supreme," or "the great terminus." The mispronunciation of the word *chi* in tai chi has become widespread and is responsible for the confusion between the word *chi* in tai chi and the *chi* that means subtle energy (described on p. 7).

Chinese Pronunciation and Spelling

For complicated reasons that would require many language lessons to explain, many Chinese words are not pronounced the way they are spelled using the English alphabet. In fact, most non-Chinese still find pronouncing the language a thankless task even after taking lessons.

None of the major systems for transliterating Chinese words into the English alphabet is very accurate. The same Chinese word or expression, such as *tai chi chuan*, may be spelled in several different and commonly accepted ways using different translation methods. This is very counterintuitive, as in English we expect the exact same word to be spelled in only one way. Chinese is different.

This is confusing to everyone except Chinese scholars who are familiar with the three most common transliteration systems—pinyin of mainland China, Wade-Giles of Taiwan, and the Yale system. For example, chi gung in the Yale system is *chi gung*; in pinyin, it is *qi gong* and in Wade-Giles, it is *chi kung*. The way the Chinese pronounce this is closest to *chee goong*—the "oo" is a sound in between the "o" and "u" of "song" and "sung." To add more confusion, neither the *chi*, nor the *chuan* of the phrase *tai chi chuan* is correctly pronounced the way it is spelled.

According to these systems, tai chi chuan is correctly spelled either as *tai ji quan* or *taijiquan* (pinyin), *tai ji chuan* (Yale), or *t'ai chi ch'uan* (Wade-Giles). However, this book will use *tai chi chuan*, which looks the least strange to Western eyes and for several decades has been the version found most commonly in print.

As a philosophical term, tai chi implies the opposite forces of yin and yang, as well as the balance and integration of the two. From many Western perspectives night–day, up–down, strong–weak, right–wrong, man–woman, etc., connote pairs that are in opposition to each other. For them, something must be either "this" or "that." From an Eastern perspective, these opposites naturally complement each other, rather than oppose or conflict, and have a common source that is beyond dualistic opposites. This source is called tai chi. The invisible quality of tai chi integrates and balances any set of opposite qualities, so they work with, rather than against, each other.

Chinese Cosmology

According to Chinese cosmology, in the beginning was the undifferentiated void called *wu chi*. Wu chi held within itself all possibilities but was beyond needing to take form. However, in order for creation to come into existence, there needed to be a creative force. This force was called tai chi.

Tai chi is inherently complete within itself, but for any manifestation of existence to function and interact with the rest of creation, tai chi needs to separate and differentiate into the opposites of yin and yang (night–day, man–woman, matter–spirit, etc.). All yin and yang pairs can be perceived either as opposites or as a complementary flow. However, both elements are partners within an interconnected continuum, with many gross and subtle relationships between them. The interplay of yin and yang was called *liang yi* by the ancient Chinese.

At a deep human level the idea of tai chi represents the capacity to balance and integrate everything within you—from the mundane to the spiritual. To implement the possibilities of tai chi you need a method—hence the fluid movements of tai chi. Philosophically and spiritually, tai chi represents personal enlightenment, a part of the universal enlightenment of wu chi.

The Meaning of *Chuan*

Although the term *chuan* literally means fist or boxing, by extension, it also means martial arts techniques, or anything to do with self-defense, warfare, or strategic encounters of any kind. At its highest levels, tai chi chuan is an exceedingly effective Oriental fighting art that was originally adapted from some of the best techniques of kung fu.[1]

The word *chuan* also implies the extraordinary physical and mental abilities that Oriental martial arts engender and are justifiably famous for. *Chuan*, when it appears at the end of a martial art's name, generically implies the specific techniques and abilities that each different martial art can pour into its followers. In tai chi's case, its specific abilities come from Taoism's chi-energy tradition, the 16-part nei gung system (this is explained in detail on pp. 226–31). These energetic abilities exist independently of self-defense movements. They equally apply to success in sports or any competitive environment, physical or intellectual.

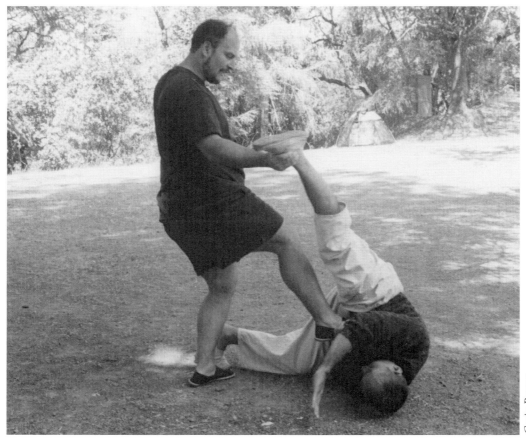

Craig Barnes

The chuan *of tai chi chuan means fist or fighting. Techniques include punches, kicks, throws, joint-locks and hitting with almost every part of the body. Here a throw and a kick are demonstrated*

[1] The development of tai chi chuan as a martial art is described in detail in my book *The Power of Internal Martial Arts* (North Atlantic Books, 1998).

Tai chi chuan's training methods are different from most ordinary martial arts, or ordinary sports for that matter. They are systematically based on the mind, energy, and intention, not muscles; sensitivity, not speed or brute force; relaxation, not tension; and a calm, still mind, rather than a violent, aggressive one. In the martial arts world these qualities give tai chi a more spiritual tone than many other martial arts. This aspect of tai chi molds and mitigates the aggression inherent in the word *chuan*.

The Integration of *Tai Chi* and *Chuan*

To implement and integrate tai chi and chuan principles, you must focus on how to optimize hundreds of important yin–yang relationships within yourself. You do this by using standing, sitting, and moving techniques in order to:

- make the body conscious. By putting the mind inside the body, you tune the mind so it becomes conscious of all the gross and subtle movements of energy within it
- separate any pair of specific yin-yang relationships into their constituent parts. This develops the potential of each part and coordinates and maximizes the smooth flow between each individual pair of opposites. The yin–yang functions are then integrated within your entire body and being, which empowers you to grow stronger and healthier as a whole, rather than just having a technique you can perform (such as chopping a brick in half with your hand)
- comprehend how internal energy or chi and the physical tissues of your body work with or against each other
- navigate the relationships between intent and manifesting chi or physical movement.

Thus, the words *tai chi chuan* have three basic implications:

1. If you only practice the movements to develop internal power (which derives from Taoist chi gung, see p. 15) without engaging its self-defense aspects, then it can be said you are doing tai chi, not tai chi chuan. From this perspective tai chi is a Chinese form of moving yoga, which is one reason for its growing appeal.

2. If you only practice self-defense techniques that do not deliberately train internal power, you are doing chuan, but not tai chi. There are about forty to fifty different Chinese martial art styles that end with the word *chuan*.

3. When both the self-defense aspects and the methods of training internal power are seamlessly integrated, you are doing tai chi chuan.

The Meaning of *Chi* (Subtle Energy)

Put simply, *chi* is that which gives life. In terms of the body, chi is that which differentiates a corpse from a live human being. To use a Biblical reference, it is that which God breathed into the dust to produce Adam. It is the life-energy people try desperately to hold onto when they think they are dying. A strong life force makes a human being totally alive, alert, and present; a weak life force results in sluggishness and fatigue.

The concept of "life force" is found in most of the ancient cultures of the world. It underlies Chinese, Japanese, and Korean culture, where the world is perceived not purely in terms of physical matter, but also in terms of invisible energy. In India it is called prana; in China chi; and in Japan ki. In some Native American tribes it is called the Great Spirit. For all these cultures, and others as well, the idea of the life force is central to their forms of medicine and healing. For example, acupuncture is based on balancing and enhancing chi to bring the body into a state of health.

Energy can be increased in a human being. Consequently, the development of chi can make an ill person robust or a weak person vibrant; it can enhance mental capacity too.

The concept of chi also extends beyond the physical body, to the subtle energies that activate all human functions, including emotions and thought. Unbalanced chi causes your emotions to become agitated and distressed. Balanced chi causes your emotions to become smooth and more satisfying. From the perspective of thought, when your mental chi becomes more refined it enhances your creativity at all levels—art, business, relationships, child rearing, etc. Spiritual chi makes it more possible for us to personally enter into higher states of consciousness, which lie at the heart of religious experience.

Tai chi, and other forms of Taoist martial and healing arts, help you develop subtle chi-energy.

Taoism—the Original Religion of China

Tai chi's parent is Taoism. Over 5,000 years old, in its oral tradition, Taoism is known for its emphasis on nature, harmony, balance, chi-energy, magic, and mysticism. Although it has fewer adherents than Christianity, Islam, Hinduism, or Buddhism, Taoism is a major world religion that continues to nourish the deepest needs of the human intellect, heart, and soul.

However, not all religions specifically heal and maintain the body's physical health or balance the energies of the body so that it does not become stressed. The Taoist tradition does—not by its poetic, inspirational texts, but through its time-tested practical applications, such as tai chi chuan, designed to implement Taoism's basic tenets.

Taoism is unique in that it is probably the only major religion in the world whose practitioners as a rule have not sought great secular power. In the past, Taoists took on such power only out of necessity to correct specific abuses. After these excesses had been corrected, they were always ready to relinquish the power and fade away, or "leave no footprints" as they put it.

Taoism has many sides to it: practical, religious, mythological, scientific, magical, and mystical. Taoist philosophy considers the outer power structure of civilization, including its politics, military power, and economics, to be fleeting and of no assistance to people in their spiritual search to find the essence of their nature. The structures of outer power simply allow us to go about the business of practical daily living with a minimum of chaos, with adequate food, shelter, and clothing. Taoists were also known as the scientists of ancient China. At that time, they were responsible for most of the nation's major scientific breakthroughs.

Being useful is a central value of Taoist philosophy—how something is useful, why it is useful, and for what. The context could be anything you could possibly conceive of, regardless of perceived value, including health, wealth, social interaction, morality and ethics, spirituality, or a tai chi movement. Practicality is the mantra. Instead of asking if you ought to be conventionally moral or if it doesn't matter, Taoists would ask "is it useful to be moral?" The answer would be yes. Rather than focusing on your narrow self-interest or the wrath of God, Taoists genuinely consider what the natural consequences are to yourself, human relations, the entire society, and spirituality if you are not moral.

The outer branch of Taoism is called *tao jiao*. Practitioners pay homage to one or many gods, visit temples where they pray, seek protection from spirits, bury their family, seek indulgences, consult mediums (especially about their ancestors), have their fortunes told, or receive other services expected from various non-Abrahamic religions worldwide. Tai chi comes from the inner or esoteric branch of Taoism, called *tao jia*. Followers of esoteric Taoism do not believe in or worship any God or gods but instead focus purely on the internal spiritual unfolding of the individual. They put the emphasis on individuals personally finding within themselves the Tao, the Body of Light, or God within. This inner esoteric tradition sees Creation's source and all its manifestations as contained within each human being. Part of the Taoists' spiritual investigation seeks to understand the ways in which the energies that compose the universe are revealed. They also believe that the mystic consciousness that underlies the universe can only be found within, by exploring the deepest esoteric and mystical possibilities of the human condition. In this sense, Taoism, by its very nature, has always been, and still is, primarily a *living*, esoteric mystic religion.

Taoism's Literary Traditions: the *I Ching*, Lao Tse, and Chuang Tse[2]

Most people know Taoism through its ancient literary works—The *I Ching*, commonly used as a divination, advice, and mathematical tool, and the elegantly written philosophical works of Lao Tse and Chuang Tse. These inspirational works also lay the practical foundations for tai chi chuan and other Taoist energy arts.

The *I Ching*

The *I Ching*, with an oral tradition going back 5,000 years, is considered to be the Bible of Taoism. It is concerned with the underlying nature and functions of all change. It also happens to be the mathematical basis of computer code, and a divination tool that untold millions of people have used to decide which way to go in uncharted waters.

Using obscure coded language, many passages in the *I Ching* are the direct source for an immense amount of technical details within tai chi. These include all its yin and yang principles, techniques from the simple to the complex, and strategies for all kinds of flow patterns within it. Equally, from the *I Ching's* viewpoint, tai chi is a way to embody and actualize the *I Ching* within the human body, mind, and spirit.

Lao Tse and Chuang Tse

Tai chi's technical details come from the *I Ching* and the classics of traditional Chinese medicine, such as *The Yellow Emperor's Classic of Internal Medicine*. Tai chi's underlying philosophical context, however, derives from the texts and oral traditions of the ancient Chinese

---

[2] Alternately spelled I Jing or Yi Jing, Laozi or Lao Tsu, Juang Zi or Chuang Tsu. *I Ching* is pronounced "ee jing" as in "jingle." The tse (or zi) of Lao Tse and Chuang Tse is a sound not found in English or most Western languages.

sages Lao Tse and Chuang Tse. Both followed the same mystical principles of the Tao, but in very different ways.

Lao Tse was the lofty, deep, and dignified sage, while Chuang Tse was the earthy, irreverent, enlightened hippie. Lao Tse had a very dignified demeanor; Chuang Tse was more like a character out of an unconventional hip television comedy with a wild and sharp theater-of-the-absurd personality and perspective. Both Lao Tse and Chuang Tse lived in a time and place where everything that comprises what we call life, be it sublime or from the gutter, was seen in the context of the sacred. Both were non-moralistic and mystical. Through the lens of what is useful, both constantly looked for emptiness and the Tao in the actions of life, rather than purely focusing on the results of specific actions.

Lao Tse wrote the *Tao Te Ching*, called in English "The Way and its Power (or Virtue)." After the Bible, it is the second most translated book in the world. Although Lao Tse passed down the broad tenets of Taoism, the oral tradition from which these principles came existed for thousands of years before his birth. His book was written 2,500 years ago during China's Warring States period. Like the world today, at that time China was in a very confusing state, well described by the famous Chinese curse, "May you live in interesting times."

Lao Tse's ideas give tai chi its incredible emphasis on the power of yin, softness, and returning to the natural easy power of a child. His timeless words are a profound vision of life on many levels. He advocated returning to a natural way of life. He saw incessant competition as damaging to society, the environment, harmonious relations, and spirituality. He looked at human conflict and war and how leaders could smooth, mitigate, or circumvent potential damage. He offered gentle antidotes to pervasive anxiety and the effects of stress on every level. He investigated the roots and proposed solutions for the lack of personal morality, and insight into loss of faith in corrupt and ineffective political, religious, and economic institutions. He expounded on the qualities of a teacher or leader and the path of patience and integrity. He felt that the more human beings want, the less they spiritually have.

Lao Tse's philosophy had a strong emphasis on personal health, longevity, and spirituality. He saw never-ending striving and not following the natural ebbs and flows of life as corrosive to health and peace of mind—especially as we age. He saw tranquility, naturalness, moderation, and keeping the innate soft quality of an infant as the foundations of health and healing. Lao Tse advocated allowing things to happen, rather than making or forcing them to occur. He likened the Tao to the empty nature of water that can be everywhere, and yet assume virtually any shape or quality while maintaining its essential nature.

Chuang Tse wrote *The Book of Chuang Tse*, the third seminal work on Taoism, and another of the major underpinnings of tai chi. While both Lao Tse and Chuang Tse emphasized the power of yin—softness and returning to the natural state of a child—Chuang Tse also emphasized developing the quality of spontaneity until it infuses all actions and becomes natural, even under the most challenging conditions. Spontaneity and naturalness are the qualities that tai chi practitioners attempt to achieve in the tai chi form and in their daily lives.

Chuang Tse's writing encompasses the most sublime mystical viewpoints, contained within a very down-to-earth style. His writing is full of anecdotes and tales, and a wicked sense of humor that strongly influenced medieval Zen Buddhists in Japan and Western hippies of the twentieth century.

Chuang Tse took the process of spirituality and the Tao very seriously, without taking the spiritual process, its followers, or himself seriously at all. He irreverently poked fun at everyone's beliefs and judgments, spoken and unsaid, spiritual and secular. Why? To help people avoid the consequences of becoming self-absorbed and rigid. Chuang Tse saw the overly serious or inflexible approach of his Confucian contemporaries as creating all-pervasive judgments that could suffocate the human spirit and sidetrack deeper spiritual possibilities, and would not reflect the true needs of life's spiritual or pragmatic situations.

As an antidote, Chuang Tse emphasized the higher calling of spontaneity and pure awareness over rigid conduct and belief, with its attendant investment in "political correctness" and a tendency to repress those who disagreed. However, his spontaneity was not based on license—do what you feel like no matter who gets hurt, and damn the consequences. Rather it was based on the spontaneity of a child, but, unlike childishness, it was rooted in deep awareness.

Taoist Energy Arts

Taoist energy arts are practical chi applications from the Taoist esoteric meditation tradition for living a better life.

The Taoists recognized that most people are not truly interested in anything beyond surface spirituality. However, many people care about things they want and perceive as useful. The Taoists reasoned that if you gave ordinary people practical chi-energy techniques that would get their needs and desires met, they would use them.

You could call these chi practices "energy arts" for living well in the world. They are termed arts because, as in all arts to varying degrees, your chi is being directed outward to produce specific effects, whereas meditation is primarily an inward-directed experience. These arts create balance within you and allow you the opportunity to gain health, peace of mind, wealth, success, and personal power. These are useful, worldly qualities that most people want.

Taoists also compassionately hoped if you practiced energy arts long enough a "wonderful accident" or event might occur where you would gain a direct spiritual perception of the potential depths of your heart and the Tao. Even if this experience was only fleeting, it still might awaken in you a real passion for spiritual realization and balanced compassionate human behavior—not because you were told to behave in this way, or because a motivational speaker charged you up, but as a result of a deeper and more genuine spiritual need that could be realistically sustained long term—meditation through the back door, so to speak. The wise Taoists said, "Give them what they want, so they will ultimately want what they truly need, realization of consciousness," whether its name be Tao or God.

After the wonderful event happens, and you delve into spirituality and meditation, the outer structure of the energy arts continues as you learn to experience ever more profound internal levels. Eventually, step-by-step, the arts lead you to what is called internal alchemy. Here the Taoist energy arts reveal their fullest possibilities.

Taoists also reasoned that even if the "wonderful accident" never occurred, at least those who engaged in the energy arts would become healthier and more balanced individuals, and live better lives. Benefiting humanity is a cornerstone of Taoism, and Taoists believe that balanced people are better able to provide long-lasting solutions to the world's real problems. They considered the time and effort spent on spreading Taoist energy arts to be well used whether or not they furthered spiritual realization.

The Taoist meditation tradition helps people attain spiritual realization by working with and balancing chi-energy, both personal and universal: hence the term *energy* or *chi* arts.

Taoist meditation has various stages and progressive energetic practices including the higher transformational practice known as "internal alchemy." These practices lead you to fully understand how within you is a tiny seed that is identical to the underlying essence of the whole universe. They allow you to realize *in your entire being*, rather than only intellectually, how the universe exists inside you and you inside the whole universe, and how to free your spirit from the limitations of the human body. It is said that through meditation you can achieve spiritual immortality in which you awaken and become fully conscious of your own soul or being.

Most people, however, aren't quite ready for this. They are not willing to commit to a task equivalent to finding the Holy Grail. When I asked my teacher Liu Hung Chieh why he didn't teach Taoist alchemy more openly, he said, "Not many people want to learn."

Taoist energy arts fall into three camps.

1. Arts that enable you to access and personally experience chi within yourself.
   These include:
   - *chi gung*
   - *internal martial arts—such as tai chi, ba gua, hsing-i, and liuhe bafa*
   - *Taoist meditation.*
2. Arts that enable you to feel chi within yourself and to perceive and work with the chi of other people, for example therapeutic energy massage, called *chi gung tui na* in Chinese.
3. Arts that do not require you to have ever directly experienced chi yourself, but which are more powerful and effective if you do. These were originally based on people's capacity to feel chi, but most practitioners today have little experience of it. Included within these categories are:
   - *Chinese medicine, including herbs, acupuncture, bone setting, and ordinary therapeutic massage (tui na)*
   - *fine arts such as painting and calligraphy*
   - *feng shui (literally "wind-water"), known in the West as geomancy. This is concerned with how the positions of the external energies of the earth, sun, sky, landscape, physical materials, color, and time can affect people, animals, and possible events. This enables you to mitigate problems, promote harmony, or create advantageous conditions in either natural or man-made structures*
   - *politics, war, science, astrology, and metaphysics.*

The question naturally arises, why so many Taoist energy arts? The answer is that a lot happens in this world and different people have different natural aptitudes, interests, likes, and dislikes which can be used to make the work of learning about chi a pleasure rather than a chore. You might want to heal but not fight, or vice versa. You might easily become drawn to and fully engaged in martial arts and painting but not feng shui or astrology, or vice versa. The more you become involved with your own natural interests, the more easily you can delve into and understand how your own energies work personally and universally.

Chi Gung

Chi gung is alternately spelled *qi gong* (pinyin), *ch'i kung* (Wade-Giles), or *chi gung* (Yale), depending on the translation system that is used.

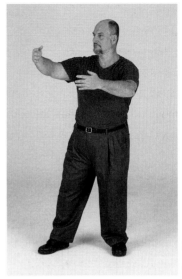

Chi gung literally means "energy work." It is the practice of learning to control the movement of the life force internally, by using the mind to direct energy in the body. Physical movements may be used but are not necessary, with standing, sitting, lying, and sexual techniques commonly utilized. Chi gung practices include many of the ancient Chinese techniques for increasing life-energy. Increased life-energy manifests itself in a variety of ways, from improved physical health to greater mental clarity and spiritual awakening. Regular practice of these exercises will lead to a body and mind that are functionally younger, so that one's "golden years" are truly golden rather than rusty.

Standing chi gung with the weight on the back leg

For more than 3,000 years, chi gung's life-giving medical and meditative techniques have benefited hundreds of millions of people by helping them achieve physical health, emotional wellbeing, longevity, and peace of mind. This "new discovery" is now being reawakened to help people in the West, just as it has for millennia in China. In our new computer age, with ever-increasing mental workloads and time pressures, we may need soft, revitalizing chi gung exercises even more than the ancients.

The Different Branches of Chi Gung

There are five major branches of chi gung in China: Taoist, Buddhist, Martial Arts, Medical, and Confucian. Each branch has various sub-schools, commonly called systems in English, and each system has sub-categories called styles, each with specific names and histories and related movement forms.

Separating out the different schools of chi gung is not so easy. In order to fully understand the functions, underlying rationales, strong and weak points, and benefits or potential downsides of most chi gung systems you are likely to encounter, it is helpful to understand clearly both the essential philosophies and methodologies of the Buddhist and Taoist systems. Often the classification and name of a chi gung method—Taoist, Buddhist, or Family system, etc.—doesn't actually describe what it does. The name in the advertisement does not guarantee its authenticity, or indicate what you will go through if you learn and practice. The words and the real goods may be different. Mixing bits and pieces of different systems often creates specific chi gung styles. The pieces of a "new style" may successfully fit together and integrate in a coherent and complete manner. Or they may fit together in a mediocre hodgepodge, which is confused or ineffective. Many "family chi gung systems" that claim to go back hundreds of years may in fact have been recently created. The story, myth, or history any given chi gung system says about itself may or may not be true. This situation is common both in China and the West.

Taoist Chi Gung

Over 3,000 years ago, meditation adepts discovered and systemized Taoist chi gung, the progenitor of all the different forms of chi gung and tai chi. They did so by going deep inside themselves. Using their powers of inner awareness, they became able to directly perceive the body's energy flows—energy channels, points, and interrelationships between the internal energy systems of the human body and its physical tissues, including internal organs, glands, sphincters, bodily fluids, soft tissues, bones, and bone marrow. These same adepts created traditional Chinese medicine, including acupuncture, healing with herbs, bone setting, and therapeutic "chi" bodywork.

Taoist chi gung is based on softness and is valued for its ability to regenerate the body, allowing you to feel and function as a young person when moving into middle age and beyond.

It is composed of 16 irreducible components, called *nei gung* by the Chinese, which means inner or internal power work (see pp. 226–31). Its methods help open the mind and calm the heart by emphasizing inner stillness, letting go, softness, and relaxation.

Although its work can be subtly intense, the trademarks of Taoist chi gung in its purest form are:

- complete relaxation of the body's muscles, tendons, and ligaments
- smooth, even, silent breathing and never holding the breath
- movements that are soft, smooth, fluid, and circular with a sense of ease and comfort
- total utilization of effort, but only to the point of not creating internal strain
- physical stretches that are accomplished by release, relaxation, and letting go of tension in the nerves and mind, instead of relying on force or willpower to push the muscles.

The Differences Between Tai Chi and Chi Gung

Tai chi and chi gung have both similarities and differences, and are often confused with each other. There is no simple way to describe the difference between the two. Appendix 1 on p. 269 sets out the explanations most commonly given and describes why these explanations only give a partial picture.

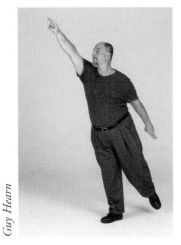

Guy Hearn

A movement from Dragon and Tiger *chi gung that would never be seen in any tai chi form*

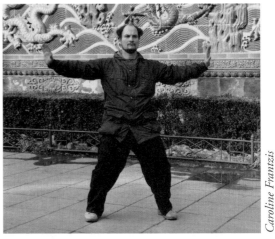

Caroline Frantzis

This movement is common to Yang style tai chi and many forms of chi gung

Conclusion

Hidden within tai chi's slow-motion movements are the gems of the accumulated wisdom of China. Its great depth is immensely useful today. It is a living, cultural legacy of the ancient world that can help you improve health, reduce stress, and make your later years richly satisfying and truly golden.

Tai chi is more than a martial art and more than most forms of exercise. It has a deep philosophical and spiritual perspective. Its gentle, slow-motion movements and sophisticated methods of systematically moving life force or chi within the body teach you to relax and open up to your full human potential on all levels—physical, emotional, mental, and spiritual.

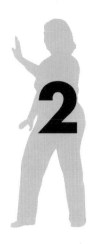

2 Traditional Chinese Medicine

The Roots of Tai Chi's Health Benefits

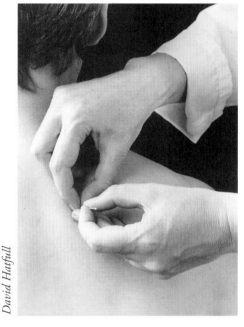

David Hatfull

An acupuncturist at the College of Integrated Chinese Medicine, Reading, UK, treats a patient. Acupuncture, chi gung, and tai chi all use chi-energy to maintain health and help prevent and heal disease

The underlying basis of tai chi as a health and therapeutic exercise originates from traditional Chinese medicine. This is why tai chi is China's national health exercise, and more than just another sport or fitness activity. All the principles of health explained in this chapter were originally used to create the tai chi forms and should be embedded within the movements. They are responsible for tai chi's potential benefits. Each health principle can be implemented in many ways using various specific practices and techniques within tai chi forms. This chapter will give you tools to assess what your health needs could be and provide a starting point to see if these needs are being met.

You can be healthy but not fit; or fit and not healthy. Or you can be both fit and healthy at the same time. In the West, people who are considered fit may be able to do 100 push-ups, run marathons, and have beautiful, muscular physiques, yet they may not be internally healthy. They may have internal organ problems (liver, kidney, heart, etc.), bad backs and damaged joints, unbalanced emotions, sexual weakness or dysfunction, or be unable to handle stress well.

Conversely, internally healthy people may be frail-looking, dumpy or fat, only able to run short distances, and not be physically strong. They may, however, have back and joints that are robust and pain-free, excellent blood circulation, and no internal organ or central nervous system problems. They may also be emotionally balanced, have the stamina to be able to do all of life's normal activities comfortably, enjoy a full sex life, and be able to handle immense amounts of stress in a relaxed way.

From the Chinese medical perspective, the first goal is to become healthy, and only then to work harder to achieve fitness, maximum competence, and optimal physical and mental performance.

In the West, health and fitness are considered synonymous. In China, health and fitness are clearly separated, especially in terms of exercise methods like tai chi and chi gung. The Chinese recognize that *health* is easily achieved by regular exercise done continuously for half and hour or less at a time, and at relatively low intensity. High-level *fitness*, on the other hand, requires a minimum of one to two hours at a session, with top performers commonly training at least four to eight hours daily.

For the Chinese, the goal of health is useful and accessible to everyone and requires less work than becoming fit. Tai chi and other branches of Chinese medicine help people of all ages to be healthy and live well to an extremely old age.

The Internal Organs of the Body

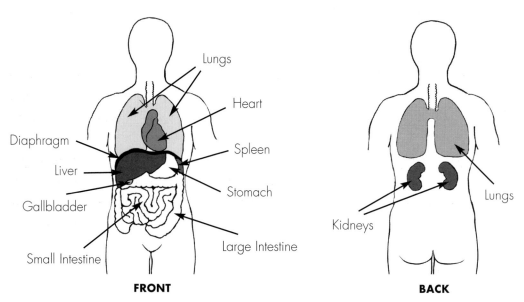

FRONT

BACK

How Traditional Chinese Medicine Defines Health

Traditional Chinese medicine sees health as more than just the absence of obvious disease. Rather, health exists when all aspects of your chi are in balance—physically, emotionally, psychologically, and spiritually. Health includes two parts: being free from organic illness or injury, and experiencing wellness—strong vitality, stamina, and a sense of wellbeing—with a clear, emotionally balanced mind. The goals of Chinese medicine are as follows:

- to achieve optimum physical and mental excellence
- to enhance longevity, so that you stay vital, mentally alert, and full of stamina as you age and remain functionally independent as long as possible
- to help cure health problems
- to mitigate or reverse the aging process
- to reduce both current and accumulated stress through energetic and meditation-based approaches to physical, emotional, and spiritual wellness.

Doing tai chi and other Taoist energy practices to achieve good health can give immense benefits to people today, just as it has done for hundreds of millions of people in China for millennia.

The Primary Importance of Chi Circulation

To maintain pain-free, optimal health, chi-energy should circulate throughout your entire body, without disruption, in a smooth, powerful fashion. The classic Chinese medical phrase is *teng jr bu tong*. If the circulation of your chi-energy is blocked (*bu tong*), you have pain and disease (*teng*). Conversely, if your chi- or life force energy in your acupuncture meridian lines is fully connected and circulating without blockages (*tong*), you have neither pain nor disease (*bu teng*)— *tong jr bu teng*. Making your chi-energy *tong* is the most basic goal of Chinese medicine and most apparent with tai chi, chi gung, and acupuncture. Balancing out and connecting your chi-energy so that it has no blockages will both get rid of the pain of disease and make you feel a whole lot better.

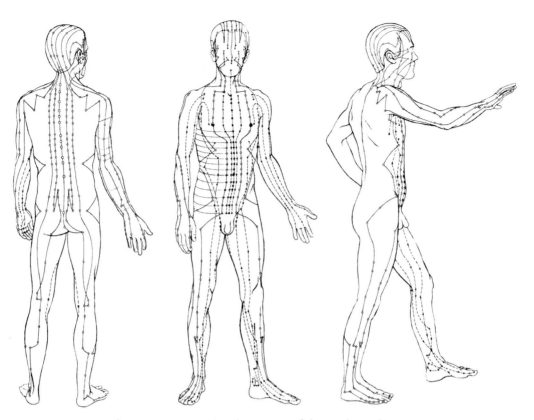

The Acupuncture Meridian Lines of the Body and Points
Along Them Through Which Chi Circulates

The Mind and Body are Composed of Chi

In the West, many people think that the body, thoughts, and emotions are separate entities. The body is real because it is physical matter, but thoughts and emotions are only creations of the mind and can be constantly changed.

According to Chinese medicine, both the body and mind are composed of chi and are controlled by the state of that chi. Chi-energy operates in the body and mind at ever more refined levels or, you could say, at higher vibrations or frequencies. Activating chi in one level affects the frequencies in one or both of the other two.

Through the medium of chi, the mind can affect the physical body for good or ill, and vice versa. Balance and smooth flow of chi in one creates balance and health in the other. Imbalance or agitated, uneven flow in one creates imbalance, discomfort, and illness in the other. Thus mental and emotional stress creates physical illness.

Physical Health

From a Chinese medical perspective, physical health begins with a lack of obvious symptoms such as overt disease, cancers, fevers, swellings, boils, broken limbs, dramatic pain, etc. But it does not end there. Physical health also requires the chi-energy of your various bodily systems to be balanced, abundant, and functioning well.

The characteristics of a healthy, energetic person are:

- reasonably rapid healing and recovery time from either health problems or damaging stress
- a lack of incipient, or potentially hidden, long-term causes of disease
- the feeling of being fully alive and vibrant during youth, mid-life and, ideally, into extreme old age
- strong and well-balanced internal organs and glands
- flexible and springy joints, muscles, and tendons
- good concentration and mental stamina.

This abundant health and energy needs to be present in all areas of your life, so that, as Chinese medicine puts it, "The chi of your body is full in all respects."

Making the effort to strengthen and balance your chi over a lifetime will produce vibrant, energetic longevity and profound wellness throughout your life. When you are younger, strong and balanced chi will enable you to enjoy life to its fullest and handle the stresses of being productive with the least possible strain. From middle age onward, a healthy lifestyle can mitigate, forestall, and combat the negative effects of aging before they take root and grow in the body.

Emotional Health

Like the weather, your emotions and psychological states have many natural environments, cycles, and moods. Humans have a wide range of emotions, which are appropriate within natural ranges but damaging when overly excessive or repressed. From the perspective of Chinese medicine, organic disease, the way your mind operates, and emotional predispositions are all intimately interconnected. The Chinese have always thought that prolonged excessive emotions easily lead to unhappiness and allow the mind to fall into morbid or destructive paths, both to oneself and others.

Psychological Health

Chinese medicine does not include a specific branch of psychiatry/psychology, whereas this is an area which Western medicine covers in detail.

For the Chinese, many common problems that we could call psychological can be positively affected, mitigated, or cured by acupuncture, herbs, etc., because they are considered generated by energetic malfunctions in the body. Deeper pathologies and malaise have traditionally been considered within the realm of meditation rather than Chinese medicine, although if severe enough they can cause energies of the body to downgrade and become imbalanced.

Spiritual Health

When Chinese medicine and Taoist meditation use the word *spirit*, they may not be speaking about the same thing (see p. 146 in Chapter 8, Tai Chi and Spirituality). In Taoist meditation "spirit" is part and parcel of *non-physical* realities rooted deep in the mind, psyche, soul, karma, or whatever one wishes to call essential spiritual qualities. Spirit's internal sources are not easily seen. From the meditation perspective, spiritual turmoil may or may not cause bodily problems, depending on a wide range of variables.

In Chinese medicine, "spirit" reflects the underlying conditions of the body's acupuncture channels and internal organs. A doctor of Chinese medicine will refer to your general external physical demeanor, energetic vitality, and the chi that generates it. Diagnostically, spirit can be observed or ascertained by investigating questions such as:

- Does the light shine in the person's eyes or not?
- Is the person's energy alive, clear, and vibrant or dull and listless?
- Is the underlying mood calm, curious, awake, and upbeat, or moody, dark, agitated, depressed, or pained?

If it is determined that the problem can be can be solved with simple but wise suggestions, or by using acupuncture needles, herbs, or chi exercises, the doctor will give them, then wait and see if this was enough.

If the physician thinks a strong concurrent factor in the patient's poor "spirit" derives from the deeper levels of the mind, in China he or she will usually consider this to be beyond their expertise, and will then recommend the patient find a reliable meditation master who specializes in these matters. This situation is similar to the way a Western doctor will refer a patient to a psychiatrist or psychologist.

The ancient Taoist meditation system has proven its effectiveness over thousands of years for healing both physical and emotional dysfunctions. In China it was not unusual for a meditation adept to also be a traditional doctor of one or multiple branches of Chinese medicine. If not, the adept still usually knew the basic principles of Chinese medicine, and the continuum between physical and spiritual illness.

These meditation adepts approached extreme emotional dysfunction in a different fashion from Western psychotherapy, which traditionally has focused on accommodating the structure and primacy of the ego. Meditation looked at emotional or mental dysfunction within the context of transcending the ego, and coming into alignment with the deeper underlying spiritual foundations of the human condition.[1] Rather than focusing on how someone should behave in society, they considered how emotions and mental functions either fostered spiritual awakening or prevented it.

The goal of relieving mental or emotional dysfunction was spiritual health. In this context, mental dysfunctions were simply seen as impediments within the complete process of becoming spiritually clear and awake—enlightened as it were. In a case of severe mental disturbance, a monastic situation with a large number of personnel was required, not just the services of a single meditation master. This is similar to the approach in the West, where for severe mental conditions a hospital with various support facilities is necessary, rather than purely outpatient services.

The Philosophy of Chinese Medicine

For over 3,000 years three words—maintain, enhance, heal—have summed up the philosophy behind all of China's potent tools for developing health and longevity, including tai chi.

Maintain

Unless you are a genetic superman, health is a gift you need to take care of and maintain if you want to keep it. As the old saying goes "an ounce of prevention is worth a pound of cure." Maintaining your health makes the difference to whether you feel well on a daily basis, or only so-so.

---

[1] The book, *Thoughts Without a Thinker* by Mark Epstein (HarperCollins, 1996), gives a psychiatric framework for this proposition from China's other major meditation tradition, Buddhism, which is much more widely followed throughout the West. As yet, most texts in Western languages focus only on the Chinese medicine perspective of the interplay between physical and mental illness. The Taoist meditation approach to issues of "spirit" has not yet been widely expressed except in extremely vague metaphorical language, virtually undecipherable to someone without extensive practical, rather than only literary, experience.

The better you maintain your body and mind, the longer they will last with little or no trouble, so that they will be a pleasure to use rather than a torment.

Enhance

The next stage of good Chinese medicine helps you enhance all your abilities and achieve optimum performance in all areas of life. This stage enables you to become exceedingly strong in all aspects—physically, sexually, emotionally, and mentally. Medicinal programs to achieve this include the use of tai chi, chi gung, nutrition, and self-massage, as well as herbs and acupuncture to strengthen and tone your internal organs.

Heal

Chinese medicine always emphasizes that it is better to keep the barn door closed (maintain and enhance), rather than chase after the runaway horses (heal). On a case-by-case basis, healing may use one or several branches of Chinese medicine in combination over time. At different stages of attempting to reverse a disease, the methods of therapy may change, especially for chronic conditions.

However, if you wish to be at peace with both yourself and the world, and feel completely emotionally, mentally, and psychically whole, you must go beyond maintaining and enhancing health and wellness, and healing yourself from specific problems. To unleash your full human potential, you need to turn to meditation and spirituality in some way that is real for you.

The Eight Branches of Chinese Medicine

China has developed eight branches of medicine. Of the eight only two are relatively well known in the West: acupuncture and the use of herbs, which each have educational institutions and national certifying boards, both in the West and in Asia.

1. **Herbs** resolve chi blockages, as they strengthen and nourish the internal organs and all bodily fluids. Like drugs, herbs are mostly respected for their healing effects; usually, however, they do not have the more severe side effects of certain Western pharmaceuticals

2. **Acupuncture** involves inserting very thin needles into specific points on the body to relieve chi-energy blockages that cause imbalances in the energy channels within us. Stimulating these points increases the chi-flow where it is insufficient, or inhibits the chi-flow where it is excessive. In the West, acupuncture is primarily known for its ability to relieve pain. However, in skilled hands it can heal the internal organs and other bodily systems just as effectively as herbs

3. **Cupping** is the placement of suction cups on the skin and muscles of the back to rebalance blood flow and correct stagnant chi. Although it is a separate discipline, cupping is also used concurrently with acupuncture and, in China, with hit medicine and ordinary massage

4. **Bone setting** is the art of setting, binding, and healing broken or shattered bones, usually without relying on the hard plaster casts of Western medical practice

5. **Hit medicine** is sophisticated first aid to heal the sprains, swellings, abrasions, and shock that often accompany car accidents, falling down a flight of stairs, or participating in sports, such as boxing or football. Teachers of traditional Chinese martial arts or kung fu schools are often fairly expert in this field. To heal the aftermath of being "hit," both bone setting and hit medicine use special Chinese medicines that look like mud. These may decrease swelling and restore functionality in a much more rapid fashion than we are used to in the West

6. **Massage**, which is called *tui na* and *an mo*, has many different schools and an amazing number of techniques, ranging from pressing acupuncture points to the manipulations of bone setters to loosening tendons, muscles, ligaments, and much more

7. **Chi gung**, energy work, consists of internal exercises (like tai chi), which may or may not include physical movement, that can be prescribed either to specifically affect a particular problem, such as asthma or nerve dysfunction, or as a general health exercise to help you maintain, enhance, and heal your health. There are hundreds of styles of chi gung, each with different exercises

8. **Chi gung tui na** (therapeutic or chi bodywork) boosts the effectiveness of ordinary massage (*tui na*) techniques by adding the use of chi (developed in chi gung) to ordinary hand massage techniques. It also has other bodywork methods that are only possible if you incorporate chi gung energy technology.

Although not a specific branch of traditional Chinese medicine, education concerning diet and lifestyle may be commonly incorporated within the treatments of all eight branches.

Chinese herbal formula for hypertension

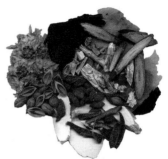

Faye Baker

Physical manipulation crosses over into bone setting, massage, and chi gung tui na. Specialists use these techniques to realign structures that have been displaced from their natural position either due to accident, poor posture, shock, weak muscles, or internal organ imbalances. Bone specialists primarily manipulate spinal vertebrae and joints, while chi gung tui na specialists work with these and other structures including ligaments and internal organs. In the West, parallel methods are those used by chiropractors and osteopaths.

Chinese medicine operates within two very different health paradigms that complement each other. In the *"we-do-it-for-you"* paradigm, the doctor prescribes herbs, inserts acupuncture needles, sets a bone, treats sprains and abrasions, puts vacuum sealed cups on your back, realigns a joint or spinal vertebrae, gives massage regularly, or projects healing energy into you.

In the *"do-it-yourself"* paradigm, patients either follow the doctor's advice on specifically what to do, such as particular chi gung exercises, how and when to do self-help medical interventions for themselves, or take up a program that includes nutrition, self-massage, and therapeutic chi-exercises such as chi gung and tai chi.

Tai chi and chi gung, without the use of external aids or substances, teach ways to use your mind to move chi-energy inside your own body. Both increase your overall healing rate (including physical rehabilitation and postoperative recovery), often reducing the time other treatments need to take effect. These sophisticated therapeutic movements overhaul, relax, and transform your central nervous system. They relieve illness and empower health by developing and integrating your body, energy, and spirit. This self-reliant approach wonderfully follows the Bible's maxim *"God helps those who help themselves."*

During different phases of resolving a problem, the emphasis may shift between different branches of Chinese medicine. Even if each of these healing methods independently could do a complete job, these shifts take into account the patient's character, mood, or lifestyle. At specific points in time some branches may be relatively more efficient, or practical, given time constraints, inconvenience, patient compliance, costs involved, etc.

Chinese Medical Principles and Tai Chi

To fully expound on the principles of Chinese medicine would require several longer and more detailed books than this one. This section will give a brief overview of those Chinese medical principles that are directly connected to tai chi. Some of the principles relate to specific pain, some to healing discernable medical conditions, and others to the general sense of discomfort and unease we all may feel from time to time.

Balancing Yang and Yin Chi

The essential point of the relationship of yin and yang to health is found in the children's story *Goldilocks and the Three Bears.* Rather than having too little or too much yang or yin, you want to adjust the mix until it is "just right."

Yin can be thought of as having the qualities of water and yang those of fire.[2] Every part of your body has both a yin and yang chi aspect to it. Yang conditions are related to dryness and heat, yin to damp and cold. Symptoms of imbalance for yang conditions can either be caused by an excess or deficiency, while yin symptoms, are mostly, though not exclusively, caused by deficiency. Both must be in balance for optimal health and wellness. If yin and yang are not in balance, the internal organs or other bodily systems progressively downgrade and become weak, sluggish, or burdened with disease. Deficient or excess yin or yang chi in one part of the body can also damage chi in other parts of the body.

Like adding or subtracting something from either side of an evenly balanced scale, problems in either the yin or yang side can tip the other into dangerous territory. Too much (excessive) yang chi weakens or damages your yin chi by burning it up and making yin chi deficient. Excessive yin can make the supports of yang chi deficient, so you end up becoming low on energy, weak in general, and prone to feeling cold. Deficient yin can exacerbate excessive yang symptoms such as a red face, anger, or dizziness.

Most severe imbalances originate with either yin or yang deficiency, for example, people wearing themselves out. When deficiency occurs, Mr. Spock's famous salute, "Live long and prosper" from *Star Trek*, could all too sadly be parodied: "Live long and suffer cruelly"—if you do live long it is without joy and with much suffering.

Tai chi has many many methods that are extremely effective in helping keep yin and yang in balance, which, from the position of traditional Chinese medicine, determines the state of your health.

---

[2] For a more detailed explanation of the qualities of yin and yang as related to traditional Chinese medicine, please refer to the excellent book written for the lay people, *The Web that Has No Weaver: Understanding Chinese Medicine* by Ted J. Kaptchuk (McGraw-Hill/Contemporary Books, 2000).

Yang

Yang chi heats you up. In the Chinese view, the stress in people in our industrial, technological society is due to people having too much yang energy. When yang is out of balance it ages your system faster and produces excess stress.

Yang chi prepares your sympathetic nervous system to gear up to meet a potentially dangerous or stressful situation. If yang is balanced, you can keep your wits about you and respond appropriately and effectively. If you overheat (i.e., if you have an excess of yang), you easily lose your temper or become manic.

If you have deficient yang, you could become incapable of doing what is needed. If yang is strongly deficient, you could lack sufficient energy to enjoy life and easily become sluggish and inert.

At the cellular level, yang heat relates to catabolism, which is the biological process of breaking down old cells. If yang is in balance, it provides the internal environment required for cells to regenerate quickly. If yang heat is deficient, the body does not clear away weakened cells fast enough. However, excessive yang heat will cause the body to break down healthy tissue, infection to flare up, and the body to age more rapidly than necessary.

Metabolic fire breaks down nutrients, either in the form of food or chi. Balanced yang helps your body assimilate and use the physical or energetic nutrients you have. Deficient yang weakens you, making you starve in the midst of abundance.

Yang heat activates your glands, powerfully affecting your bodily health and emotional states. Yang chi activates the thyroid that stokes your metabolic fires, stimulates the adrenals, which control your unconscious fight or flight response, and turns on the testes and ovaries that prepare you for reproduction. Sexual energy strongly impacts all kinds of primal instincts, and at more refined levels affects creativity and spirituality.

Yin

Yin chi cools you down and allows your body to rest, regenerate, and grow. Yin balances out the potential imbalances of yang.

Yin chi affects all your bodily fluids. Deficient yin commonly lies at the root of chronic illness. If your calming yin is deficient you easily become hyperactive and can feel like you are running on empty.

Yin chi is connected to your parasympathetic nervous system. It helps slow you down so you can keep your cool. It balances the chi of the organs so they don't overheat. For example, yin chi cools down the liver, which generates anger and is responsible for over 200 known physiological functions.

At the cellular level, yin chi controls anabolism, the process that builds up cells, helping provide the inner environment for the cells to regenerate. This is the nurturing principle of water—replenishing and cooling, and out of which all things grow. Too much yin chi and you retain fluids or become overweight or, if you do weightlifting, it may make you become excessively musclebound.

Yin chi directly affects the healthy functioning of the immune system and all bodily fluids, in particular the white blood cells, macrophages, and immunoglobins, which circulate in the blood (and saliva) and reduce or eliminate the heat of infection. The lymph system is the yin cooling fluid that collects metabolic waste (created by yang chi) and flushes it out.

You need cooling yin to regulate your glands, especially the pituitary gland, the master gland of the body that prevents many other glands from going into the red zone.

Chi and Bodily Fluids

When a stream moves continuously with a steady flow, the water stays clear and healthy to drink. However, if water becomes stagnant, sooner or later it turns putrid and becomes a source of disease. The same is true of all your body's fluids—blood, synovial (joints), cerebrospinal (vertebrae and brain), interstitial (tissues), and lymph (immune system) fluids.

Stagnant chi and fluids either pool in specific places in your body, or their flow dramatically slows down. This results in aches and pains, sluggishness, and a general sense of dullness.

Chi moves your blood. When the movement of chi gets weak enough, it causes the more serious condition of blood stagnation. As blood originates from your liver, stagnant chi and blood is associated with liver problems, as well as muscular pain and mental dysfunction.

All tai chi is extremely effective in balancing and regulating the flow of chi and the circulation of bodily fluids throughout the entire body.

The Five Elements and the Seasons

The yin–yang principle and the five elements (metal, water, wood, fire, and earth) underlie all of tai chi.

The Chinese believe the human body and the earth itself are composed of five ever-changing and circulating primal energies, commonly known as the five elements. The distinct energy of each one moves in turn to the next one in the cycle, where it then either kick starts, adds to, diminishes, transforms, or transmutes the next element. This process repeats itself continuously, moving and circulating through all five elements, *ad infinitum*. The theory and applications associated with the five elements are the basis of traditional Chinese medicine, Taoist meditation, and tai chi.

Traditionally, the way you do the tai chi form is modified to maximize the beneficial effect of each element on the body during each season. Each element is associated with a particular internal organ and a season of the year. Moreover, the chi of certain internal organs are joined together, for example the kidneys to the bladder, the liver to the gallbladder, and the heart to the small intestine.

- Metal is associated with your lungs, large intestine, and autumn
- Water is associated with your kidneys, bladder, and winter
- Wood is associated with your liver, gallbladder, and spring
- Fire is associated with your heart, small intestine, and summer
- Earth is associated with your spleen, stomach, and the period known as an Indian summer (the time between the end of summer and the onset of the colder days of autumn).

How each element directly affects you in these seasons is discussed in Appendix 2 on p. 273.

Conclusion

The health benefits of tai chi do not happen accidentally. They are based on the broader principles of traditional Chinese medicine, which has a long and successful track record. It is especially useful for chronic conditions, currently a relative weakness of Western orthodox medicine.

Based on different medical models, both the Eastern and Western approaches can complement each other to the patient's benefit. In some of China's hospitals both often co-exist in the same medical facility and are used to help patients based on their relative therapeutic and cost-effectiveness for specific conditions.

The Western medical model is based on anatomy, chemicals, and definable biological agents such as enzymes, genetic material, and neurotransmitters. The Eastern and tai chi medical approach is based on the primacy of chi-energy. In terms of exercise, tai chi does not contravene the principles of scientific Western medicine. It simply goes to the next level of effectively using chi-energy, along with sound anatomical and physiological principles.

Because of many complex interconnections, how individual or groups of tai chi moves correlate to and implement specific Chinese medical principles would merit several textbooks to give the subject full justice. In the next chapter, however, the specific section, "Give Your Liver a Helping Hand" (see p. 43), provides one example of these complex interconnections.

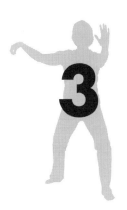

3 How Tai Chi Improves Health

Tai chi belongs to the self-reliant "heal yourself" category of Chinese medicine. It is an exceptionally sophisticated therapeutic series of exercises that helps you to feel good.

When practiced for health and fitness, the slow-motion movements of tai chi provide three basic benefits: they improve physical movement, calm and release stress from the nerves and mind, and develop chi-energy.

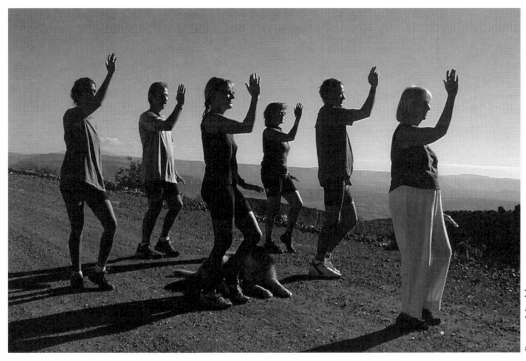

Raven Muehlgay

Tai chi practitioners enjoying the great outdoors in Jerome, Arizona

Nothing is required except to practice, ideally for between 15 and 30 minutes daily, or at least on most days of the week. These gentle, non-impact movements do not generate the potentially damaging shock, trauma, and injuries often common in more high-impact types of exercise, sports, and many kinds of dance. Because tai chi is extremely low impact, it can be done by virtually everyone.

Why Tai Chi is Done in Slow Motion

Although tai chi movements can be done either quickly or slowly, to gain the art's health, relaxation, and longevity benefits, they are primarily done in slow motion. There are many reasons for this. Most people ignore what is subliminally happening inside themselves. They were never educated to put their conscious intent below the skin and feel deeply within their bodies, much less the more subtle recesses of their mind and spirit.

Moving in slow motion enables you to consciously and deliberately access how your mind, body, and energy work. It gives you the needed time to accurately perceive and comprehend the full ramifications of what you are experiencing as you do the tai chi form.

More importantly, tai chi's slow movements slow down your neurological speed, enabling you to train your awareness to notice subtle changes and become conscious of deeper and deeper levels. Slowing down helps you become aware of and control your monkey mind—a mind that jumps from place to place without the ability to stay focused for prolonged periods in a way that allows deep concentration. As the monkey mind is tamed it becomes more and more possible for you to be consciously aware of the nuances of your unconscious mind.

If you are not aware of what needs to change, it is hard to change it. Accessing your unconscious is a first step towards making the changes that bring about the profound benefits that tai chi can give you. In some ways the human body-mind operates like a computer. Just as a computer software program automatically runs a wide variety of applications, so does your unconscious mind allow the body's anatomical functions to operate efficiently without you consciously deciding how your blood should move, nerve impulses should fire, or which muscles and ligaments to move to efficiently stretch or reach for a book.

But the code of that human software can be influenced relatively easily once you learn to access what has previously been unconscious and automatic. This is what the slow-motion movements, combined with conscious intent, enable you to do. As your awareness deepens, you recognize how to make the changes needed within yourself. You can reprogram your mind, body, and spirit to relax, to become healthy, and to be more mentally alert so that you can gain your human and spiritual potential.

Moving in slow motion also gives your body and brain the necessary time for these new patterns to stabilize within you. This allows your various bodily systems—your internal organs, muscles, fluids, and nerves—to function better. As each internal improvement stabilizes within, the link between your conscious and unconscious mind is further activated and works more smoothly.

At the basic physical level, tai chi accomplishes nine things.

1. It gives the body the movement it needs
2. It provides better support to the body
3. It massages your internal organs
4. It stretches everything inside you lengthwise, down to the smallest muscles and ligaments
5. It laterally twists soft tissues and gives you access to areas of your body, which may normally be difficult to reach and positively affect
6. It makes all the fluids circulate evenly inside your body
7. It increases chi flow
8. It increases your breathing capacity
9. It establishes (and stabilizes) highly efficient biomechanical alignments of the body.

The 70 Percent Rule in Tai Chi: an Essential Principle

A central principle that governs and underlies how you do all tai chi techniques and enables you to achieve its benefits is that it teaches students to practice and live with moderation—the 70 percent rule. The 70 percent rule lies at the heart of the living philosophy of the Tao. It is a powerful antidote to the all-pervasive stress that turns so-called success into ashes in our mouths. Above all else, the 70 percent rule helps condition the mind and body to soften and relax.

This 70 percent rule will appear many times throughout this book. Each time, it will be talked about from the point of view of how to use it in a variety of specific contexts.

The 70 percent rule states that you should only do a tai chi movement, or any inner chi-energy technique, to 70 percent of your potential capacity. Striving for 100 percent inherently produces tension and stress because as soon as you strain or go beyond your capacity, your body has a natural tendency to experience fear and to begin, even without you being aware of it, to tense or shut down in response.

At 70 percent capacity, you can throw 100 percent of your energy and effort into your practice. And by only going to 70 percent, you still generate 100 percent of the possible chi that a tai chi movement is capable of producing. Going beyond the 70 percent point in fact drains rather than increases your energetic reserves.

Staying within 70 percent of your capacities produces optimum physical accomplishment and, simultaneously, reduces psychological stress. The more you relax, the more chi-energy, stamina, and strength you will have.

The 70 percent rule powerfully counters the prevalent Western philosophy to never give less than 150 percent, as embodied in the phrase, "No pain, no gain." People who don't "give their all" are branded as lazy slackers who will never get anywhere, much less succeed. This philosophy of strain and stress helps keep our generally over-scheduled, overwhelmed society in a state of anxiety. It is a root cause of the stress syndrome, and a contributing factor to medical illness.

The core of the 70 percent rule is a creative art, not a science. It says you should use your full effort and energy, but not to the point of strain. Maintaining a natural comfort zone without using force brings the following benefits:

- It allows you to challenge your capabilities and progressively increase them without over-exhaustion, damage to your nervous system, or physical injury
- You can absorb and integrate inside yourself what you learn more easily, both in tai chi and in your life, and to build on it, ultimately enabling you to grow and flourish more as a human being
- It enables you to start storing chi, so that you have a reserve of energy when you most need it. Some stressful situations are unavoidable. Tai chi provides the reserves to cope with them and maintain that reserve under all circumstances
- Moderation mitigates against internal resistance, which is inherently a survival mechanism against excess. Internal resistance is a major reason why people can't maintain any regular exercise program, including tai chi

- The absolute amount (100 percent) of what you are capable of doing at any one time continues to increase upwards, smoothly and easily. As you reach each new pinnacle of health, strength, and stamina and continue to practice at 70 percent of your improved capabilities, you will progress in terms of absolute accomplishment, at times exponentially, without stress on your system. This gives you the will and the courage to set higher and higher goals for yourself and to achieve them.

As it is in tai chi, so it is in life. Sometimes, the improvements are so smooth and gradual that you will not recognize them until you find yourself remembering what your capabilities were like when you started. You might look back and remember that you do not get sick as often, or that you can lift heavier objects, or work harder, make decisions faster, and come home more relaxed.

Body Movement

Your body needs to move. In the same way that muscles atrophy, a body that does not move gradually loses this ability, both externally (muscles and bones) and internally (within and between your internal organs). The lack of either internal or external movement is a primary indicator of functional aging, regardless of your chronological age.

All tai chi movements are circular. They constantly rotate and twist every body part (a process often invisible to the untrained eye) in a wide variety of different ways with slow, consistent, gentle motions. These sophisticated movements continuously pull on and release structural tension from all the spots where your soft tissues (the muscles, tendons, and ligaments) insert into or connect externally to your bones, joints, and spine. Subtle, but no less powerful, pulls and releases also happen internally, allowing more movement inside and between your internal organs and related structures deep within the abdominal cavity. This improves muscle use, increases the range of motion in the joints, and gives the body a good workout.

Improved Muscle Use

Good external body movement tones and makes muscles more functional and easier to use in hundreds of ways necessary to human life. Conversely, a lack of external movement results in body pain and weakness. Tai chi's sophisticated external movements not only gently exercise the external bones and muscles but also, through subtle pressures, link all the deepest internal soft tissues inside your body.

Increased Range of Motion in the Joints

Tai chi's turns, twists, and circular movements of the arms and legs provide full articulation (the complete range of motion) to all your joints. Fully moving the joints prevents muscle pains and arthritis, improves fine motor coordination, and increases blood circulation, especially within the finer and smaller blood vessels. If your joints don't freely and smoothly move to all the angles nature designed them for on a regular basis, eventually you either "use it or lose it"—blood circulation to the joints diminishes, deposits accumulate within them, and attached muscles weaken, thereby causing weakness, pain, arthritis, and diminished mobility. Although tai chi is known to prevent, help, or reverse rheumatism and arthritis before the joints have fused, I have never known tai chi alone to completely reopen the joints after fusing has occurred.

A Good Leg Workout

Tai chi gives the legs a superb workout, increasing their circulation, flexibility, strength, and balance. Tai chi is done with your hips lowered in a slight crouch, and most movements ask that you shift weight back and forth slowly from one leg to another. This can challenge your leg muscles, increase your balance, work your lungs, and pump a lot of blood through your body.

Working the legs is critical to overall blood circulation. Upper body exercise does not cause increased blood flow in the legs as much as working the legs causes increased blood circulation in the upper body. For similar reasons, Western aerobics and other cardio-vascular exercise emphasize leg over arm movements.

Tai chi uses gravity's effect on your torso like a natural weightlifting device for your legs. This is because as you move in slow motion, one leg is continuously supporting the body's entire weight, as the other foot leaves the ground to take a step, kick, and so on. The continuous turning of the legs and waist increases blood flow to the pelvis, which enhances overall sexual capacity and stabilizes your body's center of gravity.

A Two-Stage Tai Chi Exercise for Working the Legs

In the West we often do not fully use our legs, resulting in a severe lack of strength, flexibility, and blood flow to the hip, knee, ankle, and foot joints. This causes them to prematurely stiffen or become brittle, and become incapable of providing good balance—a major problem for the elderly.

The following two-stage exercise will help you fully engage your legs. The second stage uses footwork and waist turns that are fundamental to many tai chi movements.

Stage One: Shifting the Weight Back and Forth

1. Place one leg in front of the other, with your feet wide enough apart so both could stay comfortably flat on the floor for the entire exercise. The weightless front foot will face directly forward, toes raised. The rear foot will be on a 30–60 degree angle to the toes of the front foot.

2. In slow motion shift your weight completely from the back leg to the front (and from the front leg to the back, over and over again for five minutes).

3. From time to time, progressively lower your center of gravity by letting your buttocks go down another inch or so, but do not go beyond 70 percent of your range of motion. Before the five minutes are up, you could easily be sweating. These deceptively simple-looking movements can be quite a workout!

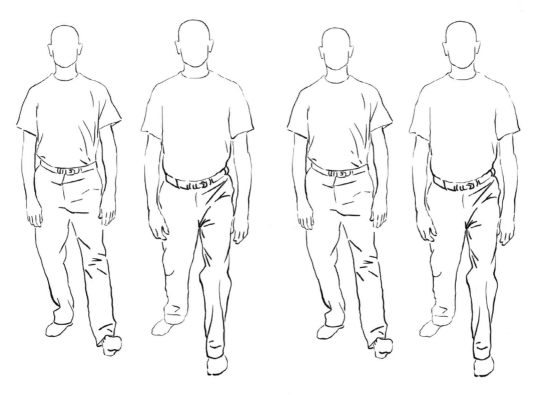

Stage One: Shifting the Weight Back and Forth

Stage Two: Adding Waist Turning and Stepping Forward to the Weight Shifting Exercise

1. Continue to shift your weight according to the three previous steps described in Stage One.

2. As all your weight shifts to the back leg, turn your waist completely to the side. (figs. b and g). When you finish, your belly button is facing at least 45 to 60 degrees to the side of where your front toes are facing.

3. As you shift your weight forward, turn your waist forward until your belly button faces the same direction as your front foot (figs. c and h).

4. If your back leg is getting tired, you can step forward until your back foot is parallel with your front foot, (figs. e and j), and then step forward with the opposite foot in front (figs. f and a).

5. Repeat this entire sequence for about 5 to 10 minutes to get a sense of the kind of workout a short tai chi form would give your legs. Keep to the 70 percent rule (see p.35) while doing this exercise.

Stage Two: A Tai Chi Weight Shifting Exercise to Work the Legs

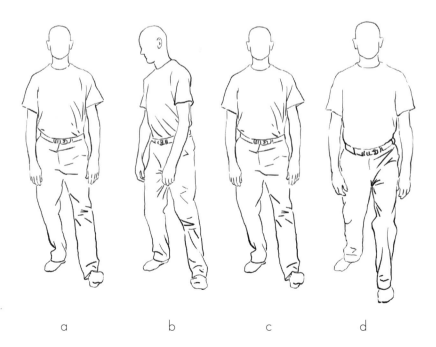

a   b   c   d

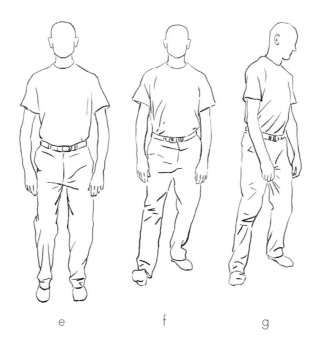

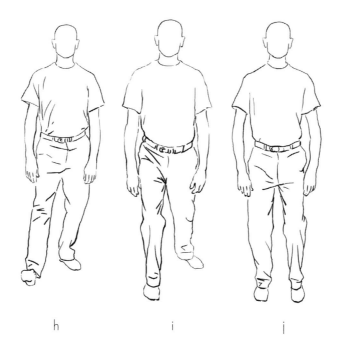

Body Support

Tai chi's movements give the body better support in three basic ways:

- By training the major ligaments which act as the springs of the body. Anatomically, the human body is kept upright by ligaments, not bones, as is commonly believed. Ligaments are also critical in keeping your internal organs from impinging on each other and thus diminishing their functioning
- By toning the muscles
- By implementing better biomechanical alignments, you are better able to give the bones and internal organs the support they need to withstand the forces of gravity that pull on all the other parts of your anatomy attached to them.

Tai Chi Massages Your Internal Organs

The movements of tai chi continuously massage your internal organs (lungs, heart, liver, kidneys, etc.). Constant turnings of the waist and limbs create gentle internal pressures that twist and beneficially massage these organs.

Taking care of your internal organs is important because your life and health depend on them. The stronger they are, the better you can perform in any area of life. Whether you are a stressed office worker, parent, or professional athlete, having your muscles massaged gives them better tone, function, and blood circulation, improves the nerve impulses, and makes you feel a whole lot more relaxed. However, in terms of health, massaging your internal organs is more important. Weakness in them and their associated subsystems can land you in a hospital, threaten your life, and dramatically downgrade what you can do in your everyday activities.

Tai chi exercises and energizes the internal organs so that they can move more freely within their natural range of motion. Tai chi's internal massage improves the movement of fluids within and between the organs and everything inside the torso and pelvis, and thus helps heal compromised internal organs. This internal massage also helps keep your internal organs in their proper places and allows necessary free movement deep within the abdomen. Otherwise these important anatomical parts (membranes, sphincters, valves, blood vessels, etc.) can impinge upon each other, diminishing their ability to function well.

Chinese chi gung and Western osteopathy share the point of view that individual internal organs have a subliminal rhythm, specific to each separate organ, which is independent of its proper anatomical placement or anatomical connections to other organs. Osteopaths call this the motility of the organ, while chi gung medicine discusses the underlying energetic rates at which body parts open and close.[1] Tai chi can regulate and positively rebalance the very subtle but important movements within specific internal organs, and make them stronger and more vibrant.

Over time, tai chi training dramatically increases your sensory awareness, so you can concretely feel and use physical tissues far below your skin. This includes ligaments and anatomical structures deep within the abdominal cavity, as well as feeling your internal organs and the energies that travel through and power them in ways the average person often cannot. Increasing your somatic awareness often makes minimal sense from an intellectual perspective, but it makes complete sense after you have been practicing tai chi for a while.

Many people have never been trained to feel the inside of their bodies. Tai chi enables you to get a new personal understanding of how your body really works from the inside out. This experiential understanding is above and beyond what standard or even progressive Western education normally give us.

Training your sensory awareness is the key to recognizing and then affecting the many energies that tai chi is capable of producing within the body. For example, the more complete meanings of "dropping your chi" or "releasing stagnant chi" require this experiential training and a good teacher to guide you through many levels of complexity until you arrive at a very simple understanding of what these technical terms in tai chi mean (see p. 59).

Give Your Liver a Helping Hand

Liver problems are quite prevalent in our society. Disease, side effects from drugs, angry personalities, excessive drinking, etc., make people prone to weak or strained livers. Even after the specific cause stops, symptoms can linger for quite a while. For example, hepatitis is particularly notorious for lingering in the body for years after the eyes cease to be yellow. I personally had this experience after a particularly nasty bout of hepatitis in India.[2] Of necessity, I became very familiar with how to use tai chi to help a damaged liver, and practiced the following technique for years. The liver is bigger than most people think and is your body's largest internal organ. Its general location is on your right side, occupying a fairly large area under and to the sides of your middle and bottom ribs (see diagram on p. 18).

---

[1] See p. 231 for more details.
[2] See foreword of my book, *Opening the Energy Gates of Your Body* (North Atlantic Books, 1993).

The technique below for giving your liver a helping hand is explained to give you a sense of how tai chi can beneficially affect the internal organs. Tai chi beginners are unlikely to encounter this method unless they are studying with someone who fully understands tai chi's health methods. Techniques such as releasing stagnant chi and sinking or dropping your chi are best learned from a competent teacher. An example of what learning about dropping or sinking your chi, (called *chen* in Chinese), involves is found in Chapter 11, p. 225.

Aside from useful but complex energy channel work, there are three essential areas to focus on when using the tai chi form to heal or strengthen your liver in general. Each mutually reinforces the other.

1. **Releasing stagnant blood and chi from the liver**. Before stagnant chi can be released, you must first stir it up so it can move and not sit like a giant lump. This can be done by making small, continuous circular movements with your arms around the liver. Do your best to feel each individual joint in your arms (especially the right one) directly connect to smaller or larger areas within and around your liver.

   As your arm joints move in circles, they generate corresponding circular movements in your liver. Large shoulder circles, for example, can move the whole liver. The elbows create sliding pressures within the liver, back and forth horizontally from the back of the ribs to your body's centerline. Your palms, wrists, and fingers can target progressively smaller individual spots inside your liver that feel stuck, hard, sluggish, or dead in some hard-to-define way. These actions can get stagnant liver chi to move. For more information on releasing stagnant chi, see p. 59 later in this chapter.

   The next two instructions are for experienced practitioners of tai chi who have already learned to feel their liver and know what it means to sink or drop their chi.

2. After you become deeply relaxed enough, you can **use your intent to release the stuck parts of your anatomy that are directly connected to your liver** and which impinge or stop each other's or the liver's movement. These could be fasciae, ligaments, valves, veins, arteries, or tangential areas, such as other internal organs. During different movements, different parts of your liver or areas nearby will feel exceptionally tight. In coordination with the bends and extensions of your arms, you micro-loosen, stretch and separate the tight areas by very gently pulling on them repeatedly, until a free internal flow and comfort returns.

3. **Dropping your liver's chi-energy down through your body to your feet**. When you have liver problems, chi-energy habitually rises up the body to the head in unhealthy proportions, often accompanied by a strong sense of heat. This rising chi can make your head feel as though it is in an angry or dissociated fog, wanting to hide or deny uncomfortable emotions within.

   The remedy is to *release and drop* your sense of liver chi down your sides, until it moves down into your lower belly of its own accord. A word of caution: *do not try to forcefully push* the chi down, or you may make matters worse by stagnating your liver's chi even more. Non-forcefully dropping the chi often produces a feeling as though your belly extends downward and is filling up. As the lower belly fills, pressure felt inside your liver recedes until eventually it stabilizes. In the case of a hepatitis hangover this could take a few months of practice; for lesser conditions, a few days, or possibly just 15 minutes.

   After successfully dropping your liver chi down to your belly, the next goal is to get your liver's chi to drop through your belly, down your legs to your feet, and from your feet into the ground.

Besides helping in cases of severe liver disease, these techniques, done within the tai chi form, often help relieve the symptoms of anger, alcohol hangovers, or severe lack of sleep.

Stretching the Body

In tai chi, stretching occurs by gently letting go of the tension in your muscles, rather than by pushing or forcing muscle fibers to stretch. Relaxing the muscles in combination with slow-motion movement gradually stretches them.

What is unique is that tai chi's movements stretch not just the large muscles, but also hundreds of smaller muscles, which most other stretching exercises rarely get to. They do so by using only normal ranges of movement that mimic activities common to daily life—squatting, bending down to pick something up, turning, or reaching out. Tai chi stretches your body using several different, yet exceptionally efficient mechanisms in combination. These include:

- smooth circular motions
- softening the quality of the mind by making the innate quality of the mind more yin.

Although this includes relaxing the mind and its background tension, softening encompasses more. The "more" is getting the quieter yin quality of the mind to penetrate your consciousness by seeping through it, and coming forward to predominate in your awareness

- using gravity to naturally and *non-forcefully* pull the muscles and fasciae of the body apart
- mentally releasing any sense of strength or tension stored in the nerves.

Tai chi's waist-turning movements stretch all the muscles of the hips, especially those around the hip sockets, the underside of the pelvis, and buttocks, which either hold up or move the spine. Continuous weight shifts between the front and back leg stretch all muscles of the legs, feet, and lower back. You can do these stretches in two ways: first externally, by making your stances either longer or deeper; secondly, internally, by relaxing so deeply that, without increased external movement, you can stretch your muscles and ligaments by directly releasing where they insert into your bones or joints. When these insertion points stretch, the long muscles attached to them naturally release and stretch.

While your limbs extend and retract, deep relaxation enables the arms and legs to gently pull and stretch all the back and associated muscles from the spine to the fingertips and toes. It also stretches the tissues within the abdominal cavity by working the interconnections between the attachments of the spine, diaphragm, and internal organs.

Reducing Pain in the Back, Neck, and Shoulders

Tai chi does a wonderful job of relieving back, neck, and shoulder pain by loosening up all the muscles of the upper body. The emphasis on flowing relaxation is especially useful for softening muscles that become stiff through long hours of working at a computer, on a factory floor, or carrying a heavy child around.

Tai chi unbinds the connective tissues of the neck and shoulders through a combination of energy work and a sophisticated method of opening up the soft tissues around the shoulder blades and within the armpits. Through all tai chi movements, the continuous motion of the shoulder blades also increases blood flow and flexibility to your ribs and upper back. This can help both your tennis and golf swings and every lifting activity your life requires. Frozen or overly restricted movement of the shoulder blades directly causes neck and shoulder pain.

The physical movements of tai chi make your back exceedingly strong and help maintain the elasticity of the deep ligaments and fasciae that hold up your entire body and spine. Improved spine support helps to relieve the causes of spinal subluxations, i.e., where your vertebrae become misaligned, causing back pain.

Waist-turning actions and deep diaphragmatic breathing soften and relax the hip and pelvic muscles, increasing the blood flow to them.

This allows the continuous downward pull of gravity to naturally open the hip sockets and release internal pressure on the sacrum (the base of the spine). This helps the entire torso to release many of the pressures and pulls it exerts along the whole spine and neck, reducing pain in the hips and lower back and improving general back, neck, and shoulder pain.

The deep diaphragmatic breathing tai chi engenders also loosens the numerous anatomical connections that extend from the diaphragm upwards to the neck, shoulders, and head, and downwards through the torso to the base of the spine and pelvis.

The 70 Percent Rule for Recovery

Tai chi can help people recover faster from spinal and other trauma, injuries, and operations. It can help speed up your overall healing rate for torn muscles and broken bones, and is often started as soon as the body can physically move or when the doctor tells you that you can begin gentle exercise. During rehabilitation, following the 70 percent rule is absolutely essential.

The 70 percent rule states that you should only do a tai chi movement, or any inner chi-energy technique, to 70 percent of your potential capacity. You should only attempt 70 percent of what you can do before you feel pain, discomfort, or any limitation in your range of motion. In order physically to heal faster and make pain go away sooner, it is important to stay within a relatively comfortable range of motion when practicing tai chi. This enables your body to heal faster and more smoothly. Finding your own 70 percent limit is an art rather than an objective science. It requires sensitivity to understand your body.

To see how the 70 percent rule works, let's look at a simple example: how far you straighten or bend your arm (and elbow joint) during spinal rehabilitation.

Spinal Trauma

If uninjured, you normally should only extend and retract your shoulder blades or your elbow joints to 70 percent of their potential range of motion.

During all connected tai chi hand and arm movements, all bending (retracting or moving backwards) and stretching (extending or moving forwards) actions, gently pull and open the soft tissues between the spine and the arms. If you are uninjured, a 100-percent extension should not cause any major discomfort, at least not more than that normally experienced by tight muscles in similar extension movements. However, to benefit fully from tai chi, such extension is not recommended.

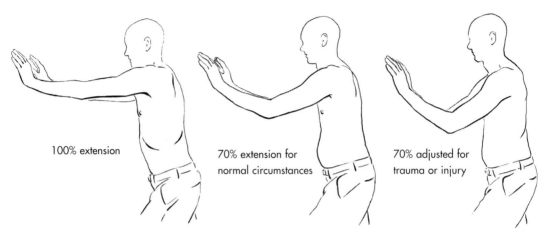

100% extension   70% extension for   70% adjusted for
                        normal circumstances   trauma or injury

The 70 Percent Rule Applied to the Tai Chi Move *Press Forward*

The situation changes dramatically if the spine is injured or traumatized in any way. Here, if you retract or stretch your hand too much, immediate pain results somewhere in your back or neck. If you exceed different ranges of motion while moving your torso or legs in a multitude of ways, at a certain point you will experience pain.

Moving beyond your comfortable range of motion (more than 70 percent) can cause pain for several reasons:

1. excess stretching for your current condition can cause vertebrae to misalign and pinch nerves
2. blood flow to the spine can become compromised
3. the chi-energy of your acupuncture meridians may become yet more blocked.

To heal an injury or trauma to your back, the criteria for determining your 70 percent boundary shifts. Your new 100 percent boundary becomes the point at which the pain begins (which may be dramatically less than what your normal, healthy 70 percent body movement would be).

Your new physical movement benchmark now becomes 70 percent of your potential range of movement *before* (not at, or after) you know the pain can start. In severe cases this could make the absolute size of your extensions and retractions, depth of stance, or height of kicks perhaps only 30 to 40 percent of normal range of movement before the injury or trauma occurred.

As you stay within the 70 percent rule, your body will:

1. maintain a comfort zone
2. not lock in the nerve and emotional memory of your trauma yet more into your central nervous system
3. cause traumatized tissues to heal and revert to a normal pre-injury state in the same or most likely a shorter time than would otherwise be the case.

Maintaining the 70 percent rule also enables you to turn an unfortunately adverse situation into a valuable resource. It gives you practical training in how to mitigate stress, rather than habitually maintaining or creating it by always pushing the envelope and going for 100 percent or more.

Postoperative Recovery

Likewise, after surgery there are often internal stitches, swellings, and reduced blood circulation to the site and adjacent areas that were operated on. Here the same 70 percent scenario applies: not at, or after, but *before* you feel the pain can start, a point which, after a few moves and stabbing pains, becomes obvious. The 70 percent rule applies not only to bending and stretching movements of the limbs but also, especially for abdominal surgery, applies to how deeply you breathe and the degree of external or internal waist twisting, which causes direct pressure to the area where you have had the surgical cuts and stitches.

Keeping to this regimen can make your tai chi movements only 30 to 50 percent as large as they were before becoming sick or injured. However this will be the fastest way to recover from the pain's root causes, allowing you, inch-by-inch, to return to your normal range of movement capacity without pain.

Pain Management

People who have been traumatized or are in post-operative recovery are often in constant, unremitting pain. Practicing tai chi within the 70 percent rule can help reduce this pain and improve recovery rates. In these cases the 70 percent benchmark becomes 70 percent of the movement range *before* your pain escalates in a clear quantum leap, for example, from a groan to a scream, or from a silent scream to a highly audible one or worse, such as doubling up in pain. This point becomes the new 100 percent. Again not as, or after, a new sharper pain level has begun, but *before*.

It has been my experience as a teacher that for many the 70 percent rule for trauma or constant pain is inherently psychologically challenging. Most egos rebel at the idea of being diminished, even if only temporarily, and consciously or subconsciously desire to immediately return to doing the full range of movements possible before the problem started. However, if this tendency can be recognized and overcome, treating medical conditions using the 70 percent tai chi rule can really accelerate your healing rate. The simple motto is "be gentle with yourself and be aware of your limitations," until you feel the injured areas of your body opening up and gradually becoming naturally comfortable rather than strained.

Recovering from Injuries

In Asia and the West, I have repeatedly seen tai chi make a real difference to how people recover from car accidents, other forms of serious physical trauma, or surgery in significantly less time than normally projected as being possible. Tai chi can also help increase the healing rate for damaged organs. However, paying attention to the 70 percent rule is essential.

I personally used the Yang and Wu styles of tai chi to rehabilitate myself after a spine-smashing car accident (the full story can be found in my book, *Opening the Energy Gates of Your Body*).

Concussion

Concussion can linger for months and cloud mental performance. The body, mind, and memory can randomly alternate between being consciously present and able to function, and feeling as though life is a spaced-out dream. For close to six months after my car accident, for example, I was intermittently forgetting and searching for information that I felt I should have known, sometimes not remembering even my own name. Tai chi increases blood flow to and from the brain, thereby helping to heal trauma there. It often regularizes the disturbed fluids and anatomical structures that surround the brain and spinal cord, such as the cerebrospinal system, that contribute to these spaced-out feelings.

The mind can forget how to focus. Some people try to tough out confused brain functions or apply more mental force to try and recover concentration. This, however, can simply turn off brain functions yet more.

Tai chi works in the sense of "softening" the brain. Gentle concentration then restarts the habit of focusing again. As the brain and head are gradually *felt* to soften, the acupuncture channels and points related to the brain begin to activate and the effects of concussion seem to temporarily abate. Just as a muscle sprain alternates between being better and worse before it completely heals, tai chi can get the felt sensations of your head and brain to soften and harden repeatedly, until you reach the point where the softening stabilizes and your recovery begins to speed up.

Whiplash

Whiplash results from a severe, wave-like shock to your spine, neck, and head as your body snaps back and forth, usually bound by a seat belt. Powerful shock causes tissues to distort with pain. Memory of severe shock can be stored either in your soft tissues or nervous system, only to painfully and repeatedly emerge later, even after specific therapies provide temporary relief.

Tai chi helps vertebrae knocked out of place to assume their normal positions, and newly restricted soft tissues to stretch back to their healthy norms. For example, besides overt muscular pain, shock can traumatize and tighten soft tissues, which can squeeze down and compromise the neck's blood vessels, with potentially lethal long-term consequences such as stroke and heart attacks. Besides relaxing and positively re-training the nervous system, tai chi also reactivates acupuncture channels compromised by the accident. These effects taken together slowly release stored body shock, keep the spine's healing process in motion, and stop the body's energy from stagnating. Otherwise, gravity's natural force can continue to strain hurt areas and gradually spread the damage.

Twisting, Turning, and Spiraling

In terms of benefits, tai chi's twisting, turning, and spiraling methods offer even more value than the lengthwise stretches that people are most familiar with. Lengthwise stretches occur, for example, if, with your feet parallel, you extend your arms and fingers far forward to stretch your shoulders and upper back. Your legs and back muscles also get a good stretch lengthwise when you are bending down to touch your toes. In tai chi, bending and extending your arms and legs can cause these same lengthwise stretches.

Twisting, turning, and spiraling continue and amplify the circular motions of lengthwise stretching. Multiple circles in your movements join into a continuous flow to create spirals. Everyone knows what it is to twist your muscles from side to side when you use a screwdriver. Your body can also make similar motions with its soft tissues so that they twist, turn, and spiral forward, like the red and white stripes of a barber's pole.

With twisting you get a two-for-one bargain. Twisting normally occurs in tai chi when you bend and stretch your arms forward, which simultaneously creates a lengthwise stretch.

Twisting and spiraling techniques are integral to all higher-level tai chi practices, from the gross to the subtle in terms of health, martial arts, energy, or spiritual work. They may be overt or hidden, but preferably not absent within any particular tai chi movement.

Twisting and spiraling encompass and amplify the more sophisticated body practices of internal stretching and circular movement. Twisting is even more important than normal lengthwise stretching for several major reasons:

- It stretches the soft tissues in a lateral, side-to-side fashion, not just lengthwise as is common in other exercises. In many ways we use side-to-side turning actions even more in daily life than simple extension-retraction movements, such as reaching or bending forward. These twisting actions significantly enhance the ability to turn the waist in tai chi, and in many sports such as golf.
- It separates your fasciae, so your muscles do not unnaturally stick together and lose their ability to move freely, which results in lost function and flexibility.
- It tones muscles in ways that lengthwise movements do not.
- It loosens and strengthens the torquing strength of the joints, such as those needed to open and close a jar or use a screwdriver.
- Most importantly, twisting opens, internally stretches, and works the tiny anatomical parts inside the abdominal cavity much more than lengthwise stretching can. This increases blood circulation within the internal organs, and releases the fasciae and membranes that bind and prevent them from moving properly. This improves the functioning of the internal organs more than lengthwise internal stretching can alone, especially in the kidneys, liver, and other organs that deal with digestion and elimination.

Regulating the Movement of Fluids in the Body

One of the major effects of tai chi is to improve and regulate the movement of all the body's fluids—blood, lymph, synovial fluid (between your joints), cerebrospinal fluid (within the spinal column), and interstitial fluid (between your cells).

This can be looked at from both a physical and an energetic perspective.

Physically, tai chi moves the different body fluids by creating a series of "pumps" within its specific movements. The pumps vary from large ones like the entire spine, belly, leg, or arm,[3] to tiny pumps within specific internal organs, joints, and between the vertebrae. As your knowledge of tai chi technique grows, your ability to activate these "pumps" becomes progressively more specific and powerful.

Energetically, the stronger the flow of chi, the smoother and more powerfully your bodily fluids move. Chi is the energetic activator that tells all your bodily fluids when to move and how. As the fluids move more, the strength of your chi increases and vice versa.

At the most advanced level of tai chi, very sophisticated methods of focusing the mind's intent will accomplish the same effects. A frequently mentioned tai chi axiom is: "mind (intent) moves the chi; the chi moves the blood (and all other bodily fluids); and the blood creates bodily strength." As you become more and more adept at tai chi, mental concentration alone will enable you to move bodily fluids in the desired manner.

Most importantly, and counterintuitively, these internal pumps do not use muscular contractions. Tai chi engages these pumps within the body by inducing continuous compressions and releases of all body tissues. This process squeezes and releases the blood vessels, enabling more blood to be pushed through them, so they can fully fill up (in sports medicine this process is called "flooding the vascular beds"). When blood vessels become fully engorged, your muscles become more flexible. The next time you take a very hot bath or sauna, notice how much more flexible you are afterwards.

These gentle pumping actions increase the grip strength—equally valuable, for different reasons, for athletes and the elderly.

Blood Circulation

Although tai chi and aerobics both improve blood circulation and cardiovascular fitness, the methods used are different. In aerobics, raising the heartbeat increases the volume of blood

---

[3] This is referred to in tai chi parlance as "the body has five bows", i.e., the spine and four limbs.

entering the blood vessels until they become flooded and pumped up. The heart muscle must work hard, often inadvisable for the elderly or those with severe medical conditions.

Tai chi increases the power of the blood vessels to expand and contract. Its internal pumping methods increase the pressure within the body's blood vessels themselves,[4] like a water-pump increases the water pressure inside the pipes of a closed system. Inducing the expansion-contraction of the blood vessels brings them into sympathetic resonance with other fluid pumps in the body (in the spine and joints for example)—just as plucking one guitar string can cause other strings to sympathetically vibrate and resonate. Because tai chi does not raise the heart-beat significantly, the movements are suitable for all health conditions.

Lymph Circulation

Improving lymphatic circulation helps strengthen your immune system. Tai chi promotes lymph fluid circulation using two mechanisms. First, deep breathing speeds up air exchange in the lungs and thereby increases the pulmonary pressure that pumps lymph along. Second, deep inter-muscular squeezing pressures inside the armpits, in the inguinal fold between the hips and the top of the thighs (an area known in Chinese as the *kwa*), and to a lesser degree at the back of the knees, mechanically push the lymph along. For a more detailed explanation of the importance of the kwa, see p. 58. Pumping actions that move lymph and synovial fluid within the joints are generated as the arms and legs gently bend and stretch.

Cerebrospinal Fluid

The motion of the cerebrospinal fluid that encases both spine and brain is regulated, maintained, and enhanced both by fluid compressions and releases, and by tiny bends and stretches of the spine and the membrane that surrounds it. These methods heal spine and neck problems wonderfully well, and produce tremendous explosive power for athletes. In order for these specialized techniques to work their best, they need to operate in conjunction with abdominal breathing and expansion–compression of the joints.[5]

Increased Breathing Capacity

Most people ignore their breath. They do not deliberately exercise to extend its duration and air intake volume. Practicing to increase your breathing capacity helps your normal breath to

---

[4] See *Vital Circuits: On Pumps, Pipes and the Working of the Circulatory Systems* by Rosemary Anne Culvert (Oxford University Press, 1993).

[5] These methods are taught in my *Heaven and Earth* and *Bend the Bow* chi gung programs.

become significantly deeper and last longer, putting a lot more oxygen into your system.

Tai chi increases your breathing capacity, regardless of whether you deliberately practice its specific breathing techniques or not:

- Sooner or later, slow-motion, even movements naturally get your breath to synchronize with them. The slower your movements, the more air you take in
- Eventually, while doing the form, your breath naturally slows to help your insides stretch, in order to bring more oxygen to the specific area being stretched. This slowing of the breath happens involuntarily. However, you can accelerate the stretching process by deliberately applying tai chi's specific breathing techniques[6]
- Your body adjusts to using oxygen efficiently. This happens through the variability of the movements themselves, which put you in a wide range of natural postures in which increased oxygen demand occurs. Because you use your natural capacities, you don't lose them.

Beginners will generally be advised to breathe from the belly and not the chest, and, if possible, never to hold their breath. Ideally, your breath should be quiet, long, and soft to help your nerves to relax, chi to flow, and your mind to become calm.

Good Biomechanical Alignments

Tai chi teaches you to align your bones and joints well so that they are correctly balanced, one on top of the other, from the feet to the head. Good biomechanical alignments enable your joints, bones, spinal vertebrae, and internal organs to move smoothly in the most efficient manner possible and with the least effort. Gravity can then flow down through them with the least muscular effort necessary, resulting in less strain on your connective tissues (ligaments, etc.).

The body has two basic mechanisms to prevent gravity making your bones or internal organs pop radically out of place. In one model, people inefficiently tense and contract muscles to hold their joints and spine together. Over time, muscular tension feels normal and relaxation abnormal, establishing a tendency for you to habitually operate in a stressed state. This becomes a problem as physical inactivity or age causes the muscles to weaken naturally.

The other model allows muscles to relax by using efficient biomechanical alignments.

---

[6] The basic breathing techniques of tai chi are fully described in twelve lessons in my book, *Relaxing into Your Being* (North Atlantic Books, 2001).

Biomechanical alignments can be thought of like a series of children's building blocks stacked within the body. In an unbroken chain from the bottom to the top, each block both supports and is supported by the blocks before and after it. Each block receives maximum support and gives maximum functionality to the other blocks.

Good biomechanical alignments provide the correct angles that help the feet, ankle, and knee joints hold up and support the hips, which in turn support the spine. Tai chi works the legs in most, if not all the angles that the body needs to support the torso's weight, thereby benefiting the spine.

Good biomechanical alignments:

- relieve pain from your muscles and bones by reducing the strain of gravity which can cause them to inappropriately grind or pull against each other
- prevent injuries, by increasing the structural supports of your body's anatomy
- heal injuries faster
- increase speed and power
- stop internal organs from being displaced or dropping excessively.

Tai chi helps improve vertebral alignments. Back pain is often caused when your spinal vertebrae go out of position. If the spinal vertebrae are in alignment and have an optimum amount of space between them, normally there is minimal back discomfort and maximum aliveness. Tai chi's gentle bending and stretching movements create an ideal vertical space between vertebrae, and, more importantly, subtly activate the spring of the ligaments that hold the vertebrae up and in place. Advanced tai chi techniques can stretch the spinal cord itself ever so slightly. This can dramatically increase the flow of energy through your nerves to all the other body parts they influence, from muscles to internal organs.

Tai chi's waist-turning actions activate and loosen all the lateral soft tissues that keep the spinal vertebrae from slipping or misaligning. Over time, the movements sensitize you to where and how subtle tensions exert pressure on your spine. This enables you to learn how to adjust your movements very slightly to release them, both when you do tai chi and when you go about your normal daily activities.

Back Pain – the Downward Cycle

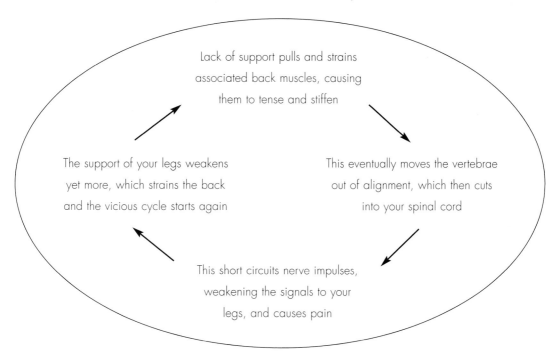

Lack of support pulls and strains associated back muscles, causing them to tense and stiffen

The support of your legs weakens yet more, which strains the back and the vicious cycle starts again

This eventually moves the vertebrae out of alignment, which then cuts into your spinal cord

This short circuits nerve impulses, weakening the signals to your legs, and causes pain

There are many even more subtle postural alignments in tai chi. The more subtle the alignment, the more specific anatomical information and sensitivity the tai chi student needs:

- Subtle alignments affect how your head and pelvis connect to your neck, spine, and torso
- The correct alignment of your torso, spine, and pelvis in turn causes your internal organs to sit in the abdominal cavity so they can most freely move within their natural range of motion
- Alignments from the spine to your toes affect the exact manner in which the bones of the feet will align with each other, an important issue for people with collapsed arches or those who wear high-heeled shoes
- The joints of the upper body (hand, wrist, elbow, shoulders, and ribs) and lower body (sacrum, tailbone, hips, knees, and ankles) correctly connect, interact, and align with each other and the spine
- Different parts of your body either lift or drop in coordination with each other.

When tiny anatomical structures are not aligned properly they create internal pressures, which block blood and other fluids from freely flowing and circulating where they should. When anatomical alignments are correct, tai chi's movements create tiny undulating actions that relieve pressure from blood vessels caused by internal structures impinging on them, allowing the blood to flow better. Increased blood flow to injured areas helps knees, ankles, elbows, and wrists heal faster. Correct alignments also increase the blood flow within deeper internal blood vessels.

The Importance of the *Kwa*

The area of the body that the Chinese call the *kwa* extends from the inguinal ligament through the inside of the pelvis to the top (crest) of the hip bones—the area around the hips where you see the bikini cut. (See the energetic anatomy diagram on p. 228.)

The kwa[7] is important for the following reasons.

1. As an alignment point, the kwa is critical in the rooting of the lower body and protecting the knees and lower back from shock. It is an essential alignment point for those with back problems or joints of the lower body.
2. It is the main energetic connection between the lower body and the torso, along the body's left and right energy channels.
3. The kwa contains the largest collection of lymph in the body, which is moved by muscular contractions. Tai chi teaches you to use the kwa to move lymph, which is one of the practice's most significant and unique contributions to health, because it helps improve the immune system.

Increased Chi Flow

The tai chi movements generate increased chi flow through the body's acupuncture meridian lines and through the channels of other energy systems in the body, such as the left, right, and central energy channels.

As a result, you effectively obtain more chi in several ways. You can unblock it, balance it, and open the flow of chi moving within and through your energy channels. Equally, increasing the flow of fluids within your body also increases the flow of chi, as they are inextricably linked.

The movements of tai chi transfer chi between the left and right hands and feet, as well as

---

[7] For more information about the kwa refer to Chapter 5, *Opening the Energy Gates of The Body*, (North Atlantic Books, 1993).

between the body's right and left energy channels. This balances the left and right sides of the body and aids in left–right brain coordination. This opens up the energy of the legs and arms more fully and cultivates the ability to absorb and discharge energy from the hands to release stagnant chi.

When a part of your body is ill or hurt, some aspect of its chi becomes blocked or pools (see p.19), and thereby becomes stagnant. Passing chi-energy through problem areas normally releases the blocked chi and gets stagnant chi to flow through and beyond its sticking points. This allows the chi to regenerate whatever damaged tissues it contacts. And as chi moves the blood, it improves blood circulation in the affected region.

China's experience has shown that using tai chi to unblock stagnant chi has been particularly useful in:

- relieving back problems
- relieving all kinds of nerve and chronic pain
- improving sexual stamina and responsiveness by opening up the chi connections between the kidneys and genitals
- helping to stave off heart attacks by freeing up important acupuncture points near the spine and behind the heart that control heart functions; this occurs through continuous movement of the shoulder blades during the tai chi form
- enhancing intellectual functions by regulating and increasing the flow of chi and blood to the brain and, just as importantly, returning it back to the body, a topic we will cover in the next section of this chapter.

How to Release Stagnant Chi

Tai chi's techniques for releasing stagnant chi includes many methods from the 16-part nei gung system, such as sinking or dropping your chi (see p. 225, Chapter 11).

When your chi becomes stagnant it either pools in specific places in your body, rotates in places where it gets stuck, or dramatically slows down.

The experience of releasing stagnant chi might go something like this. You are doing your form. Perhaps from the beginning or after a while, you begin to notice an area of your body or mind that feels stiffer, more sluggish, heavier, or more tense than other areas. Maybe you sense something in a joint, an area of muscle, something inside your pelvis or belly, or you feel a headache, or a mood of frustration, anger, sadness, etc. Gradually, as you do the form, this area's pain or discomfort progressively builds, like a movement in a symphony.

This build-up, varying from gentle to intense, is a way of letting you know that your stagnant chi is working its way through and out of your system. After peaking, the pain or discomfort subsides. This release may be either sudden or gradual. However, the difference between what the discomfort was, and the new state of ease is normally quite apparent in terms of how you experience either your physical body or psychological mood in general.

When the stagnant chi clears, the affected area feels more alive and light, and inertia seems to leave your movements. Afterward, more blood seems to flow to the previously blocked area, or tangential areas associated with it, making you feel more alive. For example, a release of stagnant chi in the hips or knees will move energy and blood down to enliven your calf and foot. Likewise a release in the neck and shoulders could temporarily cause your body sensations to become more alive right down to your fingertips or chest, and possibly make your belly feel like something is filling it. This initial sense of becoming more alive could last from minutes to hours, or become relatively stable once whatever stagnant chi was blocked has been permanently resolved.

Maybe your head feels as though it is fogged, stuck, and preoccupied, unable to let go of some particular uncomfortable or nasty mood or internal dialogue. Here, releasing stagnant chi in the brain requires a two-part process.

First, it is common to notice that one or more of the vertebrae in your neck seem slightly jammed up. Gently lift them until they separate just a little. This makes your skull lift very slightly off your neck and feel as if it is ever so slightly coming off the top of your entire spine. This will make your neck feel more comfortable and, with luck, light and airy. This will help to raise chi-energy to the top of your head, increasing and thereby ensuring an adequate flow of chi and blood to and within the brain.

Secondly, while simultaneously keeping the spine elongated and head lifted you must drop your chi and thereby return the chi from the head, down the throat and chest to the belly, through tai chi's technique of *chen* or sinking chi (which is integral to all tai chi traditions). As more and more stagnant chi drops from the head down to the belly, you begin to feel better.

Chi and the External Aura

Two basic kinds of chi powerfully affect the body. The first is internal: that which is inside your body and extends to the boundary of your physical skin. The second, often termed the aura or etheric body, is an external field in the air immediately outside your skin. If you are healthy, the outer boundary of this energetic skin may extend anywhere from six inches to many feet beyond your physical body's skin. (See the energy anatomy diagram on p. 228.) This external energetic field also is the filter through which the chi-energy of the outer environment—people, animals, natural events, power spots—affects the internal chi of your physical body. It is also the medium through which your body's internal chi and presence pushes out and affects others and the external environment.

Viewing your entire energetic situation, the chi inside your physical body is like flesh and bones, and the outer field or external aura the skin. This energetic field has been used and worked with by natural healers and psychics worldwide for millennia.

Tai chi's hand and foot movements intersect the external aura and thereby activate your internal chi without coming closer than a few inches to your body. For example, if you trace an acupuncture meridian line in the air with your hands on the boundary of your etheric, energetic skin, you activate the corresponding chi moving within that specific meridian line inside your body (this is fundamental to many medical chi gung systems in China). Every tai chi form has various specific ways to move the hands in the air, which can positively activate many useful chi patterns *inside* the body to maintain, enhance, and heal your body's chi, making you healthier and stronger in ways that may appear mysterious, yet follow predictable rules.

Missing Body Parts and Phantom Pain

Sometimes when a person has lost part of an arm or leg, or has something cut out during surgery, they experience varying degrees of pain where the missing part was, as though it were still there and wounded. By significantly extending energy past an amputated limb or through a missing lung or kidney, tai chi's intermediate and advanced techniques have been known to mitigate or stop phantom pain problems.

From an energetic perspective, phantom pain arises because even though the physical limb is missing, the energy of your amputated body part is still functioning in your external aura, as though the limb itself were still present. The solution lies in completing the body's full energetic circulation to the end of its pre-amputation physical and energetic boundaries, which may have been energetically compromised. Doing so requires very focused and refined intent. When chi flow is compromised and not circulating normally, above and beyond pain there is an even greater long-term health concern. Chi imbalances caused by the missing body part can negatively impact the circulation of chi through your body's other energy lines. This can adversely affect your internal organs and general vitality, or eventually contribute to causing a discernable disease.

Chi Flow and the Lower Tantien, the Door of Life, and the Great Meridian

In Taoism, the body contains three energy centers, or *tantiens*, located in the lower belly, the heart, and the head. (See diagram on p. 228.) In yoga, these correspond to the sex, heart, and brow/crown chakras. Taoism explains the energetic anatomy of the body in terms of three centers rather than seven or more chakras. The lower tantien is the most important energetic center in terms of physical health and vitality. It is located in the center of your abdomen, three to four finger-widths below your navel. It is a palpable energetic accumulation area and not an anatomical structure or acupuncture point, and as such it must be felt rather than visualized. The size of this energetic accumulation varies between a tiny pellet and a grapefruit. In many higher-level practitioners it can create a noticeable "chi belly," even in extremely thin people with minimal body fat.

The lower tantien is the only energy center that connects all the major and minor energy channels that continuously circulate around your body and that specifically affect every aspect of your physicality. Ideally, the lower tantien smoothly pulls all the body's major energy circulations into itself. Then it unites the chi, speeds it up, and thereby diminishes whatever stagnant chi is present. Finally, it propels the accumulated chi out into the body once again to circulate through all the channels of your system.

The lower tantien acts like a battery or dam, storing energy for future use. When you complete a tai chi session, energy circulates though all your channels, and returns to the lower tantien at the end. There, a drop of chi can be deposited and stored until the chi accumulates and becomes a great reservoir. If you accumulate more chi through practicing tai chi than you use in your daily life, you create an energetic "savings account," which can be drawn upon in times of emergency, illness, or high stress. Having stored some chi, it is there for you when you need a boost, and ensures you don't exponentially deplete your energy reserves when becoming exhausted. This gives you a much better chance of returning home neither grumpy nor totally exhausted on particularly hard days. The more chi stored, the more you can maintain a high level of health, enhance your performance abilities, heal yourself, transmit chi from your body to heal others, or hit a golf or tennis ball better.

All tai chi practices consider a person's capability to store and generate chi from the lower tantien to be key to successfully obtaining the physical benefits of developing chi. The lower tantien is at the center of Oriental martial arts, healing, and meditation practices, because practitioners believe that it is the energetic source that makes us either feel fully alive, vibrant, and strong, or weak, depressed, and ineffectual.

Directly associated with the lower tantien are two other important energetic components—the door of life (*mingmen* in Chinese), and the great meridian (*dai mai*).

The Door of Life

The door of life is located directly behind the lower tantien on the spine. It is called the door of life, because it is directly associated with the kidneys, the internal organ regarded as the source of life-force energy (see diagram on p.18). A direct energy channel internally connects the lower tantien to the mingmen, and as such it is often nicknamed the back tantien.

The Great Meridian

Chi-energy spreads from the lower tantien in circles. The largest circle is called the great (*dai*) meridian or energy channel (*mai*)—or dai mai. It is one of acupuncture's eight extraordinary meridians. When the lower tantien's chi connects to the door of life, it starts a powerful energetic circuit that encircles the waist. Equally, the waist turns performed during tai chi serve to activate this energy channel.

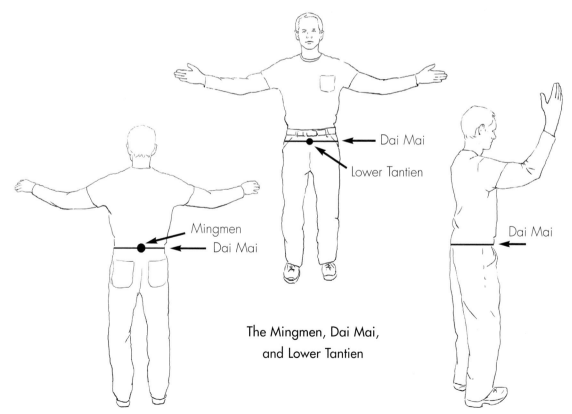

The Mingmen, Dai Mai,
and Lower Tantien

If you consider the tantien as the center of a wheel lying horizontally, the great meridian is the outside of the wheel. It connects all the vertical acupuncture lines in the body, transferring chi between them.

There is a connecting energy channel within the body between the lower tantien and the door of life to the great meridian, and chi travels between them in both directions. This enables energetic movement in the great meridian to travel via the door of life through the connecting channel to activate the lower tantien. Likewise, in the opposite direction, via the mingmen and the great meridian, the lower tantien balances all the acupuncture lines, which are energetically responsible for many of the physical functions of the body.

Beside strengthening and balancing many of the primary energies which affect the internal organs of the body, working the great meridian also helps the lower tantien to store energy. Techniques to develop the great meridian are an essential component of all acupuncture meridian line chi gung systems and tai chi.

Conclusion

Few health exercises have stood the test of time for as long as tai chi. The practice of tai chi has been steadily growing in the West for decades and its benefits are mostly spread by word of mouth. Those who do tai chi know it makes them feel and function better.

This low-impact exercise can do as much or more to improve overall health and relieve stress as aerobics and other exercises. It improves muscle use and the circulation of blood in your cardiovascular system without generating potentially damaging shocks or trauma to the joints and organs. It keeps everything inside you healthy, from the smallest muscles to ligaments, joints, bodily fluids, vertebrae, and internal organs. Besides giving you a good whole-body workout, tai chi helps you to reduce and manage pain of all kinds, and to recover more rapidly from trauma.

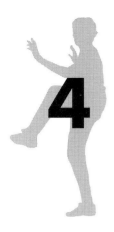

4 How Tai Chi Reduces and Manages Stress

The ability to let go and relax in all ways—physically, emotionally, mentally, and spiritually—is at the philosophical center of Taoist practices and the core of all tai chi. *Relaxation allows happiness to flourish; tension diminishes this possibility*. Tai chi, and other Taoist energy arts, are deservedly famous for their ability to compensate for the downsides of stress and promote relaxation on progressively deeper levels.

Few Westerners have ever experienced complete deep relaxation and its qualities of calmness, awareness, and inner balance. Tension is so normal that we are psychologically unprepared for the fact that physical relaxation can be a living reality, rather than a mere metaphor.

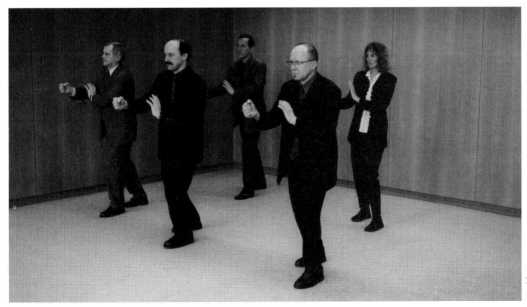

German executives practice tai chi for stress management

Rolf Werner

All too often, fatigue and lethargy are confused with relaxation. So many people are stressed out that most can't remember ever having felt their body be fully relaxed. Typically, many top athletes or dancers, when asked to relax their shoulders, neck, and chest, cannot—even after a life spent in physical training.

Tai chi trains you to feel progressively more deeply inside your body. With tai chi practice, you develop an awareness of where your body holds tension within itself, and this gradually extends into your daily life. You begin to notice how your neck and shoulders tense when working long hours at your desk or computer, what happens inside your body when you are angry or sad, or how mental exertion under pressure causes your body to fatigue.

From the perspective of stress, the techniques of tai chi are more about training your central nervous system than your muscles. It is jangled nerves that lie at the root of anxiety, particularly in our technological age, with its immense amount of intellectual output. This anxiety affects almost every population group—from babies to the elderly. Overloading the brain directly affects your nervous system, resulting in a fight or flight response that induces tension and causes the nerves to overload. Over time, this can produce a condition in the brain and nerves, where almost any thought or decision, no matter how small, causes anxiety.

The regular practice of tai chi teaches you to consciously relax your mind and body before it starts to tense, and prevents the condition from being painful or chronic. Because chi moves through the central nervous system, the process of relaxation begins by smoothing out the functioning of the nerves. Relaxing the muscles is only part of this process.

The regular practice of tai chi trains the body to relax at increasingly deeper physical, emotional, mental, and spiritual levels through the interaction of five components that are embedded within its movements. Tai chi:

1. trains the body to practice moderation, by implementing the 70 percent rule
2. increases your level of chi-energy, thereby strengthening the nervous system. Weakening the body's chi can cause the mind and nervous system to become agitated. Conversely, an agitated mind and nervous system can downgrade the body's chi, eventually resulting in physical problems
3. empowers your general level of health and stamina. It also releases and flushes out stress and illness-related toxins from your body and mind. Whenever you feel a major release of toxins, be sure to drink lots of water to help release the toxins faster, and to help prevent them from being reabsorbed into your system

4. stretches and elongates tissues which habitually become shortened or congested due to stress

5. creates an environment where your mind can reduce its jangled, congested, and churning thoughts and experience a clear, open, and relaxed mental space.

Tai chi practice develops the habit of allowing the sense of inner pressure to pass and be replaced by a sense of inner peace. It is tai chi's synergistic approach that gradually releases stress—no one single component is the "magic bullet" for learning to relax deeply.

Practicing Moderation: Tai Chi's 70 Percent Rule

Tai chi's greatest challenge for Westerners is learning the timeless art of moderation. Tai chi's philosophy is moderation in all things: never doing too much or too little. Moderation allows your body and mind to relax and easily absorb the fruits of your efforts, to integrate them inside yourself, and to build on them. By doing so, you can be as productive as possible without setting yourself up for chronic stress and all the physical and emotional problems that accompany this. From tai chi's perspective, moderation is essential for us to reach our full potential—without burning out, succumbing to internal resistance, and letting stressful behavior become habitually ingrained.

Tai chi trains moderation through the 70 percent rule, which was introduced in Chapter 3 (see p. 35).

Striving for 100 percent inherently produces tension and stress because as soon as you strain or go beyond your capacity, your body has a natural tendency to experience fear and, even without you being aware of it, begins to tense in response.

Moderation mitigates against internal resistance, which is inherently a survival mechanism against excess. As you become more stressed, your nerves begin to develop resistance against doing what is needed as a biological, self-defense mechanism. This mechanism is subliminal; however, when you override it by not adhering to moderation, your level of stress snowballs exponentially.

High Performance and the 70 Percent Rule

When you are going for high performance, if you push yourself too far from your comfort zone, at a certain point, even though you feel like you have accomplished more, you actually become less and less productive. This is very counterintuitive for people who have embedded stress and "going for the burn" into their lives in order to become high achievers. Convincing them that moderation will benefit their training sometimes only occurs after they have injured themselves and are in pain.

For example, if you push yourself too far in athletic events, you progress more slowly even though you feel like you are working harder, and you court more training injuries. Often, the time it takes to recover from training injuries becomes longer. By working just a little less, your peak athletic abilities will arrive sooner and be sustainable longer. Moderation will help you perform better.

High performance tai chi presumes that you have been practicing for more than an hour a day for over a year, have passed beyond what is required of beginning students, can stay within 70 percent of your physical and mental capacities, and have a dramatically acute sense of where your limits lie. If you only have average ability and are practicing for less than 30 minutes a day, you must stay within the 70 percent rule.

Once you are willing to practice within 70 percent of your physical and mental capacity, you can extend that capacity to somewhere between 80 percent or, at most, 85 percent. This is because you have begun to understand where the fine line is between further productive gains and starting to reduce performance.

To even attempt going from 70 percent to 80 percent presumes you are extremely fit in your tai chi practice. If you are going to go a tiny amount above 80 percent it is important that your internal awareness of how your body is adjusting to this extreme strain is very acute and precise. Otherwise, do not go past 80 percent, and under no circumstances exceed 85 percent, or there will be a price to be paid in terms of long-term productivity.

The Dynamics of Relaxation

In China, the Taoists discovered that physical relaxation is only the beginning of relaxation's potential. There is also the need to relax your chi-energy, emotions, and mental activity and discover what it means to you to be a spiritual being. Complete relaxation integrates all these kinds of relaxation.

Working with the body, tai chi uses five outer and inner qualities to encourage relaxation.

1. The outer form movements provide a container through which you can recognize where tension and stress is lodged inside your body and mind. We have not been trained to be aware of, nor to consciously relieve, these levels of tension.
2. Slow-motion movements give your mind the time first to recognize, and then to exert conscious effort to change a host of specific interactions within your body, chi-energy, and emotions. Moving too quickly—physically or mentally—causes many to miss these interactions.
3. The form helps chi to flow smoothly and powerfully, promoting relaxation with full awareness.
4. Tai chi trains you to focus your awareness inside your body so that when you try to release a specific point of tension with your mind, your body will listen, attempt to obey the suggestion, and finally relax. Most of us have not been trained to know how to put our mind and intent deep within our body through to the bone. Tai chi provides the training environment where this can occur.
5. Tai chi trains you to focus chi-energy and the mind's intent into tense emotions and thoughts until they relax. The more tai chi has a spiritual orientation, the more this mind-training process is engaged.

Physical Relaxation

Many people have never experienced deep muscular relaxation. All too commonly, Westerners are trained to maintain muscular tension. The body has over 600 muscles, with their associated soft tissues. Because the muscles of most people are habitually tense and contracted, we easily become numb to muscular sensation. We don't even feel our small muscles, and may rarely use the smallest ones. Even directly after good sex and the release of orgasm, some level of residual tension remains. If tension does go away, it is only for a few fleeting seconds or at the most minutes. Although muscle relaxants can help reduce gross tension, many times the relaxation they produce makes people feel as though their bodies are not really relaxing, only that the pain is not as bad.

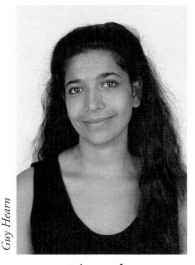
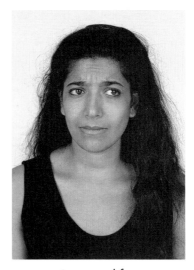
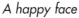

A happy face   *A stressed face*

In the beginning stages of tai chi, deep physical relaxation sneaks up on you. Only for a moment at a time does your body let go and become soft and open. To many it is a revelation, a true surprise. Initially, deep relaxation comes for short periods, and then disappears for a while. Relaxation seems to have a mind of its own. You cannot predict its comings and goings.

As you continue to practice, your muscles noticeably soften. Your body begins to give you unambiguous feedback about the degree to which your muscles are relaxed or not, both in a variety of positions and while maintaining complex physical movements. Once you begin to relax the body's surface muscles, you progress to relaxing its deepest recesses such as your internal organs, spine, and glands.

Over time, tai chi provides deep physical relaxation, a stable foundation from which you can become neurologically and emotionally relaxed.

Neurological Relaxation

One of the ways chi-energy travels though your body is within your nerves. All good training in tai chi strongly emphasizes relaxing every nerve in your body. By relaxing the nerves, muscular relaxation can go deeper and become a permanent part of you, rather than being just an intermittent, fleeting experience.

Deep neurological relaxation is more profound than muscular relaxation. It is an antidote capable of healing the all-pervasive damage that anxiety and stress produce, and it increases both physical and mental stamina, making you more productive than heaps of caffeine ever can.

As relaxation deepens, your nervous system starts to run more smoothly, making physical coordination and athletic prowess easier to come by. This well-kept secret lies behind the potential effectiveness of tai chi as a fighting art, and easily translates to all high-performance physical activities. A fast moving, smooth running, fluid nervous system can easily generate physical speed and power, and translate thought into action with minimal resistance.

Emotional Relaxation

As your nervous system opens up and loses its resistance to change, tai chi begins to help you gain access to, and let go of, the nastier emotions that tear up your insides—hatred, jealousy, self-pity, greed, inappropriate anger, etc. Maintaining emotional negativity requires tension that can destroy much of life's joy.

A relaxed muscular and nervous system provides the required support base that your new, more open and free emotions can live and thrive in. Releasing the physical tensions in muscles, organs, tissues, and your nervous system provides the support to relax emotionally and maintain a tranquil inner world.

The body's most powerful sources of negative emotion reside in the internal organs—the liver, kidneys, lungs, etc. (see Appendix 2, p. 274). Emotional relaxation requires that you use your mind and all the chi that you can generate with tai chi movements, to focus your intent and gradually diminish the binding forces within those internal organs that feed your emotional tension. Relaxation can now develop varied yet subtle subjective qualities, which both improve your moods and help turn you into a more positive force in the world.

Tai chi will help lay a foundation of inner relaxation and stability, from which you can permanently release your negative emotions and exorcise your inner demons. Otherwise, out of habit and lacking any positive alternatives, emotional negativity will simply return.

How Tai Chi Can Help Overcome Anger

Tai chi can reduce the tensions that lead to outbursts of anger, help you calm down and let go of your anger, and mitigate damaging physiological hangovers.

Getting really angry makes you very tense. In turn, unrelenting bodily tension helps maintain ongoing anger, leaving your body in a perpetually angry state and ever more prone to anger. If you reduce your body's overall tension level, you can overcome many of the major physiological triggers to becoming angry in the first place.

Whether you are the person who is angry or the person who is receiving the anger, your mind races, your heart pounds, your blood pressure rises, your breathing becomes erratic, your muscles tense, and your stomach clenches. From a Chinese perspective, the consequences of explosive anger include your acupuncture points becoming blocked, an increase of stagnant chi—especially in the liver (in Chinese medicine, the liver governs the emotions of anger), and a release of toxins which makes you feel like your insides are being poisoned. You need to get rid of these toxins so that they do not continue to overwhelm your body and mind. Tai chi can help you reduce and clear out the effects of anger by shifting your body out of a fight or flight response, and allowing the body to recognize that it does not have to release stress hormones any longer. It gives you something to do that helps you avoid feeling helpless. Focusing your mind on something that takes up your concentration gives less space in it for anger.

As you do tai chi's rhythmic, slow-motion moves and exercise your large and small muscles, your physical level of tension drops and allows more blood to flow through your body. Your heart will relax as your blood pressure drops. Your chi starts to flow more smoothly through your whole body, helping your internal organs to return to a normal state. Your nerves begin to quiet down and normal breathing patterns resume. Slowly, but surely, your mind begins to quiet down as you focus on your movements, rather than on what triggered your anger. Finally, you consciously allow the energy of your anger and liver to dissipate and move down and out of your body, ensuring that you release this energy completely rather than letting it become stored in your liver, ready to flare up at the next provocation. (See Chapter 11, p. 225 for an example of one kind of progression in chi development.) As your liver chi drops, your body begins to dissipate the chemical messengers inside your system which otherwise leave you feeling poisoned inside.

For some, visualizing yourself using tai chi's fighting applications (see Chapter 7) as you do the form allows you to release your anger safely and helps you feel you are actively doing something to release it. This helps you to become progressively more neurologically relaxed.

Practiced on a regular basis, tai chi relaxes and gives you the equivalent to taking a stress-reducing vacation. After vacationing on a beautiful, isolated beach, where you experience a quiet, restful, and soothing lifestyle for a while, you find you don't get tense and angry so easily. Rather than lashing out if somebody says or does something unpleasant, you tend to just shrug off the potential slight without it ruining your day. Tai chi can provide a calmer, more balanced mental environment.

Doing tai chi after an outburst of anger can help resolve these problems and flush the toxins out of your body.

Finally, if you are in the middle of an outburst of anger, practice tai chi and after a while, as your chi becomes smoother, it will become possible for you to let go of your anger. This is a better solution than kicking the dog or disturbing the peace of your family and friends. And if the anger is caused by a nasty turn of events or a seemingly unsolvable problem, by doing some tai chi you can get some internal space (previously occupied by the anger) to find creative solutions, rather than rage or brood.

Mental Relaxation

Stress usually causes the mind to speed up, often uncontrollably, and to have jangled, disassociated thoughts—what the Chinese refer to as "the Monkey Mind." The more you relax, the more your conflicting thoughts begin to slow down and lose their force. You begin to see things with more clarity and less frustration.

Mental relaxation helps:

- your mind to settle and become calm, allowing you to focus on what you are doing
- your mind to multi-task without mental tension and distraction
- connect your brain to your body without strain
- you to retain awareness of single or multiple thoughts without becoming tense and feeling yourself pulled in different directions
- insights and ideas to emerge naturally.

Tai chi helps you to experience the extremely subtle tensions that exist between your spinal cord, internal organs, and brain that produce corresponding tensions in the mind. Letting go and relaxing these tensions requires great sensitivity and starts you down a road where it becomes increasingly difficult to blithely ignore your personal self-delusions or those of others. For many, letting go of the mental tensions that bind is infinitely more useful to everyday life than tai chi's effects on physical abilities. Being able to think with clarity and not have your thoughts churn and jangle your nervous system provides a profound sense of mental ease.

Doing tai chi to let go of mental tension is also extremely important in terms of health and longevity.

Mental stress and the desire to be perfect are linked. Many people seek to do tai chi's movements perfectly. But the Taoist concept of tai chi does not demand that you learn the movements perfectly. It asks only that you apply some effort, learn at your own pace, and improve. *Seeking perfection keeps you stressing about the future, rather than relaxing into the here and now.* Mental relaxation requires you to focus on the journey rather than reaching a "perfect" destination.

Many people beat themselves up mentally and emotionally when they invariably fail to be perfect in what they do. To paraphrase an old Taoist saying, "Gods may be able to be perfect, fully grown mortals cannot."

Energetic Relaxation

Most Westerners do not relate to the concept of energetic relaxation and tension. Relaxation causes chi to flow smoothly and fully. Tension causes chi to flow erratically, in a jerky, spasmodic manner and with significantly less power. When chi moves smoothly, it has a natural balancing quality that helps the body to regenerate. The smoother the chi flow, the stronger and healthier the body becomes. That is why people can be simultaneously relaxed and strong. Gradually it becomes obvious that when your chi flows smoothly, relaxation follows it like a shadow, and vice versa.

According to the ancient Chinese, an overly active or agitated mind "can eat the chi of the body," running the system down and potentially resulting in all kinds of disease. Tai chi provides you with the means to get the buildup of excessive chi out of your brain and back into your body and internal organs where it belongs. With relaxation, the chi in your acupuncture meridian lines flows smoothly. If the body is tense, you develop blockages.

Energetic relaxation goes deeper than muscular or nervous system relaxation. When it occurs, it happens in some indefinable way unique to each person, as all of us have a unique experience of what it feels like to inhabit a body comfortably. When profound energetic relaxation happens, your body truly lets go, until, without qualifications, it feels that all is as it should be. Internally you feel healthy and without blemish.

Understanding the Effects of Tension and Chi Blockage

Some people notice that when they become anxious and stressed, their stomachs clench and churn or their shoulders and necks become tight. In the West, we commonly say they are "uptight," an accurate word for how the tension of the mind and emotions affect the body.

Stress attacks the weakest part of the body, causing muscles, ligaments, and tendons to tense. The flow of chi becomes constricted in the weakest places of the body and, if the constriction continues, those weaknesses will increase and move on, attacking the next weaker place in the body.

An easy way to understand how the dynamics of tension affect the body is to do the following exercise.

Make a fist with one hand. Tighten your fingers as much as you can. Try to hold this position for five minutes, but stop if you feel too much discomfort. Commonly, this is what you may experience:

1. You will feel a certain amount of physical discomfort. It is hard to hold a fist in tension for a long period of time. Tension is uncomfortable and takes a lot of energy to sustain

2. Your fingers and knuckles may turn white. This is because the fluids (blood and the synovial fluid in the joints) will flow out of them—and so will the chi

3. The muscles and connective tissues contract and shorten. Tensing anything tightens muscles and ligaments and binds fasciae, connective tissue, etc. Over time, tension makes it progressively more difficult to lengthen and release the muscles and connective tissues

4. The discomfort in the hand may begin traveling up the arm. The forearm begins to feel tense, then the upper arm. Then you may feel discomfort in other parts of your body that you tend to tense up: shoulders, jaw, etc. Tension tightens up the whole body

5. You may begin to experience negative feelings ("Why did this author make me do something that feels so uncomfortable?"); or it may bring up other unpleasant thoughts. Tension causes the nerves to rev and negative emotions to well up

6. If the tension has traveled to a place where chi has been blocked for some time, besides physical pain, you may experience the associated negative emotional feelings that caused the initial blockage.

So far you are just holding tension for a few minutes and feeling its results, not just in the fist, but also in other areas of the body, emotionally and mentally. In reality, this is very similar to what happens inside the body when tension builds up and you do not release it. The chi also becomes clogged and the fluids stop circulating at particular parts of the body. The part of the body that is most clogged progressively weakens and can become diseased.

Now open your fist. You'll feel tremendous relief ("Whew! I'm glad that's over"), and notice:

1. The discomfort in other parts of your body dissipates
2. Negative emotions dissipate
3. The blood and other fluids flow back into your hands and fingers (though it may take up to ten minutes for the hand to feel normal)
4. The fasciae and muscles stretch and you can fully move them again.

Relaxation revives the ability of the body to stretch and retain flexibility.

Spiritual Relaxation

The practice of tai chi may turn you towards meditation and spirituality. You may begin to gain the true strength and confidence to attempt to relax the obstacles that have bottled up truth, honesty, faith, kindness, generosity, love, and whatever other qualities may be stunted. These obstacles prevent the full flowering of your soul.

If your heart is sincere, tai chi can be used as a focal point for relaxing the mind–body shackles that bind your "soul" or "inner essence" and through which you experience the human condition. Tai chi at increasingly subtle levels will help you examine your emotional demons, thought processes, subtle perceptions, and your acceptance of what is possible to change or not, as well as your desires and attachments, both positive and negative, your sense of identity or self-worth, and your relationship with your innermost essence or soul.

Only you can decide if this may be something good and useful for you. The most useful potential of spiritual relaxation, according to the Taoist meditation aspect of tai chi, is to relax into your being, or to relax your soul. To the best of my knowledge, tai chi does not conflict with the practices or beliefs of any religious faith. Regardless of your specific religious beliefs, there is an old saying which seems to be universally appropriate: "If you take one step toward God, God will take two steps toward you."

The Dynamics of Stress

The term "stress" is constantly seen and heard in modern society. It means many things and conceptually is often used to describe multiple scenarios and experiences. It may be caused both by external influences and by inner personal, emotional, and physiological ones. What someone feels and means when they say that they are "stressed out" varies greatly from person to person.

East and West both agree stress is killing us, although each has different perspectives as to how and why. Tai chi and the Eastern view see the roots of stress lying in weakened and unbalanced chi-energy. Western science views the problem in terms of various destructive biochemical or genetic interactions.

Few escape stressful situations in the West, particularly in our fast-paced, technological society. The common complaint from all sectors of society is the feeling of being overwhelmed—by excessive information, the strain of balancing family and work, and political and financial problems. Asia's economic powerhouses are also stress-ridden, and people have the same unrelenting work pressures as their counterparts in the West. But while tai chi is commonly used in the East as an effective stress management tool, it is less common in the West.

East and West have different ways of looking at the dynamics of stress. But even though they may approach stress from different directions, their conclusions are the same: chronic, unmitigated stress causes the body to weaken and become prone to disease. Both agree that some level of stress, no matter how small, is unavoidable. Stress is the price we pay for being productive, for getting the difficult, necessary, things accomplished and for surviving extreme circumstances.

What is important is how you deal with stress so that it does not become chronic and uncontrolled. If you succeed in this, when a real need arises your stress levels rise, but only for long enough to deal with the situation that is presented, and you recover relatively quickly. Your mind and emotions then need some quiet and regular intervals of tranquility in order to rest and heal your nervous system and thereby allow your body to regenerate.

As mentioned earlier, the ancients found that an overly active or agitated mind or brain "can eat the chi of the body," resulting in all kinds of disease. They found this especially true among intellectual workers like imperial bureaucrats, who enjoyed a relatively high standard of living but became burned out relatively young. In order to recover from stress the Chinese considered four commonsense pre-conditions to be necessary:

1. Deal with daily affairs without massive habitual emotional swings, whether overt or suppressed below the surface

2. Have regular intervals of relaxation and tranquility during workdays, and make them significantly longer on days off
3. Get regular exercise, either gentle or robust
4. Sleep in a way that is regular, deep, complete, and restful.

Losing the balance between rest and activity can and does act like corrosive acid. It tears down the chi of the body, affecting your emotions and ability to focus and think clearly.

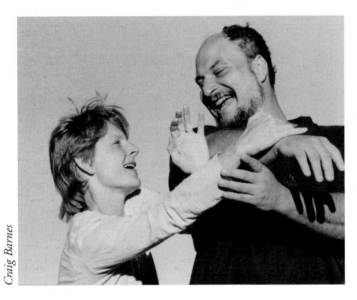

Craig Barnes

When Push Hands *is practiced in a playful, non-threatening manner, it can be a wonderful antidote to stress.* Push Hands *is the bridge between tai chi form work and sparring*

Besides physiological consequences, chronic stress also has potentially detrimental behavioral and emotional side effects. These may include the adoption of diversionary tactics and coping mechanisms such as tobacco, drug, and alcohol abuse, and various psychological disorders, including insomnia and depression.

The Eastern View of the Downward Stress Spiral

From the physical to the spiritual, the Eastern view looks at stress cycles from the perspective of chi-energy. To get things done and withstand life's difficult moments, you must use up some of your body's chi-energy—physically, emotionally, mentally, or spiritually. The more you are required to put out a massive and prolonged amount of energy, the more stress you undergo and more chi-energy you must expend to deal with it.

You regularly acquire a given volume or amount of chi-energy daily by various methods, for example eating, exercising, breathing, living right, doing tai chi, etc. Doing tai chi before your day begins is a positive way to acquire some of the chi-energy you need, so you feel better and more energized on a day-by-day basis.

You can also squander and deplete your chi. Examples of squandering chi include engaging in excessive and draining strain (perfectionism, not resting or going to bed when exhausted), destructive and addictive pleasures, having continuous emotional outbursts (anger, sadness, etc.), and churning the mind obsessively. You may recognize that these stresses and strains can wreak havoc and drain you, but you cannot seem to stop.

Your chi reserves were primarily created and accumulated while you were in your mother's womb, and are called pre-natal chi by the Chinese (or a strong or weak constitution by the West). Core reserves are drawn upon to provide the chi-energy to deal with the most severe forms of chronic stress: life-threatening illness, serious physical or emotional trauma, and multi-year, unrelenting work pressure with intolerable hours. After enough energy has been used up and some of your core reserves are lost, your normal vitality slips and downgrades, destroying your quality of life, and making you more vulnerable to illness and injury. Once your body is in a habitual state of chronic stress, you are required to expend extra energy just to keep the stress from dramatically escalating and causing breakdowns. Otherwise it is difficult to experience a fully comfortable and vital daily life.

In the short term, the practice of tai chi helps the body to save and store chi and thereby mitigates and counters the losses that are activated by chronic stress.

1. Saving chi compensates and makes less disagreeable any potential damage caused by acute stress factors: missing a night's sleep, short-term colds or illness, or bumps and sprains, etc., thereby ensuring these events only cause temporary grief and suffering, and don't kick off a negative downward stress spiral with long-term negative health consequences
2. If unused, short-term stored chi makes you feel better on a daily basis
3. Whatever chi-energy is unused gets transferred into your core reserves—your body's long-term chi-energy savings.

In the long term, the practice of tai chi will store chi in your core reserves and help you deal with life-threatening illness, serious physical or emotional trauma, or unrelenting work pressures. Core chi reserves are difficult to increase except, for example, by taking a year off, or by deliberate training in energetic methods like chi gung or tai chi.

How the Downward Spiral Works

The downward spiral nastily, endlessly, replays the question, "What comes first, the chicken or the egg?" If your body's chi-energy weakens, your mind gets stressed out more easily. Agitated thoughts and chronic stress cause your mind to never completely wind down, which tears your body's energy apart. As your energetic bank account increases (by doing tai chi for example) you get fewer symptoms of stress. Conversely, when your internal chi-money supply is depleted the hard times begin or get worse.

Constantly at work, your mind compulsively and relentlessly churns over various thoughts or emotions. This causes excessive chi and blood to get stuck in the head. This in turn blocks the optimum circulation of chi through your energy channels and the return of blood from the brain to the heart necessary to re-oxygenate it. Over time you lose your ability to release your internal strain.

Internal strain progressively saps your chi, and the loss of vitality and general inability to cope creates the subtle conditions for physical disease to occur.

In Chinese medicine, psychological manifestations of stress are considered as being either yang or yin chi symptoms. As your chi further degrades, it first becomes difficult and then nearly impossible to control your predisposition toward violent emotions. These powerful emotions could have outward yang qualities such as an explosive temper, raving, snapping, greed, anxiety, and paranoia. Or they could manifest as inward yin qualities such as depression, lack of confidence, melancholy, an inability to follow through, a sense of all-pervading helplessness, or feeling a lack of control.

A constantly emotionally agitated mind unbalances the chi of the body, causing strain to the internal organs that easily results in different kinds of disease. In the Chinese view, long-held negative emotions damage specific internal organs. For example, fear damages the kidneys; anger (either active or passive) the liver; giddiness and hysteria the heart; grief and melancholy the lungs; and worry and indecisiveness the spleen. These in turn result in specific diseases, which may have the same or different names as those of Western medicine.

The Negative Stress Cascade

As stress chews up your chi it initiates a progressively negative cascade of events that deplete the internal organs:

- Your body and nerves seem to get sluggish. You now have to push and continuously summon up the effort to accomplish things, rather than it being fairly easy and effortless. Energetically, your blood circulation and kidneys are coming under pressure
- Your nerves and general awareness seem to be engulfed in a cloud that requires real effort to penetrate. Stress is straining your kidneys (the source of your life force) and disrupting the smooth blood flow to and from your brain. If you become much more easily distracted and the fog thickens, your spleen is weakening
- Your nervous system feels strained most of the time. You want to rest but can't. You push yourself forward either with a sense of no joy and drudgery, or by becoming hyper or, in the worse cases, manic. You now start to unconsciously snap at others, or suffer in silence with a sense of seething resentment. Your nervous system is beginning to shred, and your liver and heart chi are taking strong hits
- Your immune system weakens. It seems that minor illnesses like flu and colds visit more often and linger longer. The chi movements of your bodily fluids, including lymph, are losing their steady, even, regular flows
- At this juncture, stress begins to snowball as its effects become chronic. As with any condition, if you now take remedial measures you can reverse or prevent the weakening of your body functions from becoming uncontrolled.

If you do not take remedial measures, the negative cycle now seriously escalates:

- Your nervous system seems to progressively speed up and rarely slow down. Inside, there is a constant internal rev like that of a car ready to go from zero to sixty miles an hour in a few seconds, or the jangle of drinking too much coffee. Stress is now beginning to affect and strain the chi-energy of your glands, especially the adrenals. This internal rev is an indication that stress is, metaphorically, beginning to harden and congeal inside your body
- Your sleep patterns downgrade and become irregular, so that you never feel fully rested. Your emotions become more erratic as the fluids of your cerebrospinal system begin to

release all kinds of potentially unpleasant hidden subliminal memories. You may or may not be consciously aware of them, but you do react to them and often find yourself going on emotional roller coaster rides for seemingly no reason. The emotional stress adds yet more strain to all your bodily systems, especially the nerves and internal organs, making your chi yet more erratic. Thoughts seem to scatter as though they have their own free will. Your ability to focus plays a peek-a-boo game. Now it's there, now it's gone and you don't know when or why. You begin to take longer to do the same things. You easily lapse into protracted internal dialogues or daydreaming without being able to control it. You begin to explode or seethe at the slightest provocation and often become fixated on being right. The chi flowing through your nerves is beginning to cause them to no longer regularly fire smoothly or communicate well with your downgrading internal organs

- Sleep becomes fitful. Even after getting a full night's sleep for several nights in a row, you still wake up tired and can't shake the feeling all day long. Your kidneys and liver are under severe attack. Your nerves are now in a constant state of chronic stress, creating pain in all your muscles, especially in the back and neck. Vertebrae easily go out of alignment. The rev in your glands rarely turns off, exhausting them further. You sense you are aging inside, regardless of your actual age or energetic starting point

- Vicious reinforcing cycles are now in play. Even after a weekend with plenty of sleep you still don't feel rested. Your kidney chi is severely weakening. Your connective tissues, ligaments, and fasciae are either becoming too loose or too tight. Soon they may not provide the necessary full anatomical supports for your muscles, bones, joints, and internal organs. Your joints may begin to ache as the chi within their synovial fluids ceases to function and pulse properly. The downgrade of all your internal organs continues. As a result your glands increase their rev, potentially damaging them, while straining and draining your internal organs and nervous system yet more

- Even if you regularly go to the gym, the weakening of the connective tissue results in your insides feeling like they are becoming more stiff and brittle, and just waiting for minor injuries, which begin to occur more often. Parts of your body feel less alive. Blood is ceasing to fully circulate to affected parts, which begin to tire or hurt more easily with minimal usage. Blood pressure problems commonly follow

- Your chi is becoming exhausted. You have trouble keeping things together. If this continues long enough you may be setting yourself up for severe illnesses, such as chronic fatigue syndrome, a nervous breakdown, severe chronic back problems, or a heart attack.

The Western View of the Dynamics of Stress

While the term "stress" is used frequently by the general public, a scientific consensus on the word's meaning does not exist. Within the scientific community stress has become a very hot topic of research. The relationship of chronic stress to disease has received a great deal of scientific attention in recent years and continues to be actively studied. Considering the constantly stressful lives of many people in the modern world and the links between stress and disease, it is surprising that most of us are still able to function without succumbing to a stress-related disease.

According to Western medicine, the body responds to emergencies or stressful situations by evoking the stress response—a series of behavioral and physiological processes—including the release of several chemical messengers (hormones) into the bloodstream. The initial stress agent may have many sources, including physical trauma such as an accident, hunger, extreme heat or cold; personal endangerment such as a threat of violence; or psychological stress from financial problems, work-related pressures, or difficulties in personal relationships.

Within seconds of exposure to the stressor, the sympathetic nervous system is activated. This component of the stress response is commonly called the "fight or flight" response. This response is vital to escape from immediate threats and to act quickly and decisively in emergencies. Activation of the sympathetic nervous system results in enhanced secretion of the chemical messengers epinephrine and norepinephrine (also known as adrenaline and noradrenaline).

There is a second, slower set of events which takes place within minutes and involves increased release into the bloodstream of a group of steroid hormones called glucocorticoids (GCs), primarily cortisol in humans. Glucocorticoids have many actions throughout the body that are primarily of a catabolic nature.

During the stress response, the heartbeat's strength and speed is increased to enable enough blood to be pumped and shunted to the areas that most immediately need it, such as the brain, heart, lungs, and limbs, and away from less immediately crucial areas. Increased blood flow helps deliver energy nutrients to essential muscles and organs, and improves mental acuity in emergency situations. Stress hormones also help increase the amount of glucose available to meet the body's increased need for energy during stressed periods. Bodily processes such as growth, reproduction, and digestion are often suppressed during stress. This is because the body views them as energetically expensive and non-essential to survival in emergencies.

As opposed to the life-saving effects of hormone levels during periods of acute stress, chronic stress and continual hormonal release may have very detrimental long-term effects on health.

This is the primary reason why chronic stress is often considered to be the leading cause of disease in our society.

Many important bodily processes are negatively affected by long-term stress including (but not limited to) glucose metabolism, musculoskeletal health, growth, tissue repair, and the functions of the immune, cardiovascular, reproductive, and neurological systems. Chronic activation of the stress response has been linked to many disease conditions including hypertension, osteoporosis, ulcers, diabetes, atherosclerosis, impaired growth and development, reproductive dysfunction, and irritable bowel syndrome. Some people experience significant amounts of discomfort or pain without discernable origin, a secondary symptom to muscular tension.

Chronic stress also has psychological consequences, including insomnia and depression.

Here are some other physiological effects of chronic stress highlighted by Western medical research and science:

- The eventual onset of diabetes. Chronic elevation of cortisol results in increased mobilization of energy stores and increased production of glucose leading to elevated blood glucose concentrations
- Continual mobilization of glucose can also lead to the eventual atrophy of healthy tissues and fatigue
- Stress hormones, including cortisol, have been shown to cause an elevation in blood pressure and have been clearly linked to hypertension. Hypertension can in turn damage the heart, blood vessels, and kidneys
- The immunosuppressive effects of stress hormones may result in increased susceptibility to infectious diseases
- Chronically increased levels of stress hormones suppress memory
- Muscle weakness. A primary effect of cortisol on metabolism is the reduction of most of the body's protein stores, except from the liver, both by decreasing the amount of protein being made and increasing protein breakdown in cells. With chronically elevated hormone levels, muscles can become so extremely weak that a person may not even be able to rise from a squatting position
- Increased susceptibility to osteoporosis. Overabundant stress hormones decrease the accumulation of calcium in bones and deplete the bone matrix
- Stress has also been linked to stomach and small intestine ulcers. Many ulcers result from the presence of a bacterium called *Helicobacter pylori*, which causes inflammation of the

gut lining, rendering the gut cells unable to protect themselves from ulceration. Many people have these bacteria, but don't develop ulcers. Stress has been shown to worsen the ulcer-causing effects of the bacteria because the body's immune defenses are lowered, thereby allowing the bacteria to flourish. A group of chemicals called prostaglandins, which are believed to help repair damaged gut walls before ulcers develop, are decreased during stress

- Stress can contribute to infertility in women and reduced sperm production, premature ejaculation, and impotency in men, partially through inhibition of the reproductive hormones.

In our fast-paced, high-pressure society, people are constantly bombarded with stress on a daily basis that can continuously activate the "fight or flight" response. This can lead to persistently high circulating levels of stress hormones and subsequent pathological consequences. For these reasons stress is often considered to be the leading cause of disease in the West today.

Type A Personalities: Preventing Burnout and Increasing High Performance

Many successful athletes, doctors, lawyers, politicians, and industry executives, commonly called Type A personalities, are particularly susceptible to burnout. These people are highly competitive, and often aggressive and intimidating. They push hard to achieve their goals and do not often slow down. They can be emotionally explosive.

These qualities tend to burn out chi and cause stress to snowball, particularly as Type A people get older and their nervous systems and glands move into a high rev that is chronic and destructive. This expends life-force chi in very wasteful and inefficient ways and prevents people from increasing, or even maintaining their high performance capabilities well into their old age.

Some people were born with the incredible genetics to withstand this kind of drain on their chi-energy. They can push hard, barely sleep, carouse or work for days on end, scream and have temper tantrums incessantly, smoke a few packs of cigarettes a day, survive their heavy alcohol or drug habits, and still outlast us all and live to a hundred. As an old saying goes, "They give ulcers rather than get them." However, most people can't live this way and remain healthy.

Adding tai chi to their daily routines and learning the 70 percent rule is an excellent antidote to the downsides of Type A life styles. Tai chi shifts the Type A tendency to always push energy out into more relaxed and effective new patterns that increase high performance.

Tai Chi and Mental Health

In cases of mental illness, tai chi is not a substitute for qualified medical, psychological, or psychiatric treatment. However, tai chi can positively improve people's mental health. Besides relieving many stress triggers that contribute negatively to mental health, tai chi is particularly useful in other mental spheres. It brings people back into their bodies rather than being purely "in their heads." On a lesser level this helps reduce neurotic tendencies, so life can become more than a series of intellectual games.

In more serious cases, tai chi can give current or potential mental patients some very necessary mental space. This space enables them to separate two important things: first, really feeling their body; and second, thinking thoughts. This avoids the confused situation where people with mental problems might have thoughts about how their body feels, yet in reality may either not be feeling their body at all or may have inaccurate perceptions of these body feelings. This confusion can have obsessive or destabilizing effects resulting, for example, in anorexia nervosa, obesity, or feeling hallucinations within your body.

Tai chi has been used to re-establish a positive psychological body image after major physical traumas such as car accidents. It does so by reorienting a personal mental image toward how well the body functions, and how that can be increased. This positive mental image helps combat the natural tendency of many people to obsess over what their body theoretically was or should be, which easily leads to anxiety or depression.

Why Healers Need Tai Chi

The life force or chi-energy is transferable between people. This is why one person can heal another and why people enjoy being around charismatic individuals or people in love. Their life force moves into you and makes you feel better. The opposite is also true. People do not relish being around sick, depressed, manic, or other kinds of "draining" people, who can suck the life force out of you and tire you out, making you lose the pleasure of living. From a chi-energy viewpoint this creates problems for professional healers with close one-on-one human contact with clients or patients.

Healers in the caring professions (doctors, therapists, social workers, clergy, etc.), or professionals with large amounts of human contact, such as teachers, need to learn how to renew and manage their energy effectively over the long haul to avoid becoming drained and progressively less effective. These skills are especially critical for therapists who have prolonged one-on-one contact with very draining and needy people in pain. The Chinese call this energetic transference, giving out your psychic "blood." Sick people need balanced energy; it is because they do not have it that they become sick. However, the Chinese also recognize that when the healer's life-force chi-energy is drained significantly, his or her healing abilities diminish. This is no less true for massage therapists and chiropractors, who transfer energy with their hands as it is for homeopaths, psychologists, intensive care nurses, and psychics who give their emotional, mental, and psychic energy to others.

Tai chi and all Taoist chi-energy practices can give you practical ways to increase your personal energy, stamina, and resistance to, or recovery from, burnout. As long-term stress reduces success in your job, doing some sort of energetic practice daily, or at least regularly, is advised.

In China, it is considered wise to take the time, every day, to do some kind of chi practice which can replenish the human life-force energy the therapist continually gives out to help others. For some, a half-hour a day is enough; others with exceptionally heavy client loads might at times need up to two or three hours a day to replenish their life force to a satisfactory level. Energetic training teaches healers how to pace themselves internally, and recognize when they are exceeding their individual energetic limits. If you lack some sort of regular energetic metronome, it is often almost impossible to recognize when you are going over the line before it is too late.

Tai chi's standing and moving techniques drain negative energy from your body that you absorb from patients and clients during the day, as well as build up and replenish depleted energetic reserves. Opening and closing techniques (see p. 231) work very well for releasing jammed joints, or re-stretching a body which may have shrunk because you may have unconsciously patterned the bodies of your excessively contracted clients.

Tai Chi and Post-Traumatic Stress Disorder

Tai chi has been used to help reduce post-traumatic stress disorder. It has been used by Veterans Administration hospitals to deal with Vietnam vets who have suffered traumas from physical injuries and psychological dysfunction. Memories of war situations get locked in the body and metaphorically harden there. This makes it difficult and immensely time-consuming to fully release the traumatic memories through counseling or other therapies. Tai chi's physical and mental relaxation techniques help soften these "body memories" and reintegrate these two interconnected kinds of trauma. By helping the body let go, tai chi gives the mind space to also let go and allows the traumatic memories to become more malleable and accessible.

The patient can then move from being closed down and resistant to becoming more open and available to the benefits of therapy. This makes the therapist's job easier and quicker. As the hardened memories stored in the body become more plastic, the easier it becomes to find solutions within the patient's mind.

Conclusion

Tai chi is a consistent program for learning patience and moderation. The absence of these fundamental virtues causes us to exceed our individual human limits and create tension and stress.

The effect of the accumulation of stress in the body can be thought of in terms of a snowball. As a snowball runs downhill, each new revolution increases it to many times its original size. The larger the snowball that you start with, the faster its absolute size grows. However, if you catch the snowball early on, you can reduce the speed by which it grows.

The best way to mitigate the increasing volume of stress is to regularly reduce it so that you start, metaphorically, with a smaller and smaller snowball every day. Tai chi helps dissipate and reduce the growth and final potential size of the stress snowballs that come from really major life traumas, such as deaths, illness, job loss, divorces, bankruptcy, etc. Not mitigating the snowball's size makes it harder to recover and get on with your life, sowing very dangerous seeds for the future.

Tai chi conditions you to decrease your stress snowball:

- through the subtle learning process of how to do this art
- through regularly doing the movements
- by engaging in the other aspects of tai chi, including push hands and spiritual pursuits.

Being physically relaxed makes it easier to have a happy or positive attitude. Just adding a little extra practice time daily can be extremely beneficial. In the short term, tai chi can reduce the time it takes for the immediate physical discomfort and emotional pain to heal from significantly stressful events, such as a major fight with a close family member or friend. Long term tai chi practice can reduce the potential final size and future growth of the stress snowball that remains after the natural time needed for the pain to heal has passed. This helps prevent a chronic stress hangover, which can linger, grow, and maintain the wounding effects of the original event's pain long past its normal time. In this way you avoid laying one major level of stress on top of another.

For tai chi to work, you must practice a reasonable amount every week. To gain tai chi's benefits, you must do the form, not just think about it. Doing the tai chi form:

- cools down and relaxes your nervous system
- mitigates the drain to your chi reserves that the stress snowball normally eats into
- replenishes the chi that stress drains from your ordinary and core reserves.

Learning and doing the tai chi form mirrors the complex choices of modern life. The ancient yet still relevant art is a humbling exercise in obtaining emotional wisdom. You can only do what is possible, no matter how much more you desire. Finding patience and moderation balances out and reduces the negative sting that is often inevitable to get necessary things done. Tai chi consistently trains you to recognize what is possible within our capability to be productive at the present moment without becoming stressed out, as it allows you to achieve physical, emotional, mental, and spiritual relaxation.

5 Tai Chi and Longevity

Longevity—the practice of living well into old age—makes tai chi and all the Taoist chi arts justifiably famous in China. In the ancient world, virtually no other major culture poured as much energy and enthusiasm into considering the implications of longevity as did China. One of the country's enduring cultural and mythological heroes is Peng Tsu who, according to the imperial archives, lived for eight hundred years.

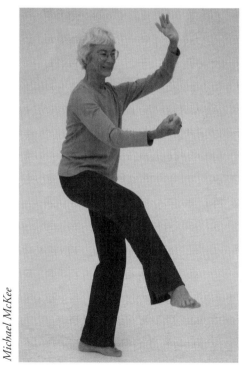

Michael McKee

A 70-year-old practitioner demonstrates balance and flexibility executing the Yang style tai chi movement Step Forward, Parry and Punch

The traditional Chinese medicine principles of maintain, enhance, and heal, introduced in Chapter 2, have created the longevity regimens that have been trademarks of Chinese medicine and all Taoist practices, including tai chi, for thousands of years:

- Maintaining the good health of your mind, body, and spirit means not just being free of disease and pain, but brimming with stamina and vitality.
- Enhancing your physical, emotional, mental, and spiritual functions helps you realize your full human potential.
- Healing helps bring your physical, emotional, mental, and spiritual self into balance.

Achieving the goals of the maintain, enhance, and heal principles are the major reasons older people do tai chi. This is not to live a thousand years (which was an obsession of China's ancient culture generally, and some Taoist alchemists specifically), but rather to retain and live in the complete fullness of your physical, sexual, and mental faculties for as long as you can.

The exact day of our death, of course, is one of life's basic mysteries. Living well until that day arrives is entirely possible. Tai chi can make the difference between merely coping with and enjoying life—between watching your grandchildren play and actively getting out and playing with them. Tai chi helps you fundamentally change your internal environment so that life becomes wonderful to live and not a burden to be carried around. It is an exercise that will constantly challenge you; a self-exploratory tool to help you till your internal garden and make what is ordinarily hidden in life become obvious.

From my own experience, two of my teachers, Wang Shu Jin and Liu Hung Chieh, were amazingly strong, physically flexible, and extremely alert well into their seventies and eighties. As a student of tai chi studying all over China in my twenties and thirties, I remember meeting many ordinary practitioners of great age, whose physical strength could give me a run for my money.

Wang Shu Jin, one of China's great internal martial artists, always credited his robust health to his chi practices. During our first meeting, he said to me, "I can eat more than you, I can have more sex than you, and I can fight better than you, but you call yourself healthy. Well, young man, there is a lot more to being healthy than being young, and it all comes down to how much chi you have."

I studied with my main teacher Liu Hung Chieh when he was in his late seventies and early eighties. Although Liu looked like a man in his seventies, the shine in his eyes, his

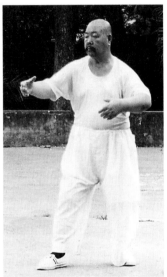

Bruce Frantzis

Wang Shu Jin, at approximately age 80, doing standing chi gung

physical movement, and mental stamina were the same as someone in his prime. Liu taught and poured energy into me for three and a half years, for between three and six hours a day, seven days a week. Once or twice a year, his physical functions and mental stamina seemed to dramatically downgrade for a short period. His natural physical and martial arts movements slowed considerably; his joints stiffened; and it became difficult for him to speak and act quickly with strength for prolonged periods. His face looked increasingly tired and hollow, and the shine went out of his eyes. I had to walk very slowly so he could keep up. He would then give me homework and ask me to let him be alone for a few days or weeks.

When I returned, he had completely regenerated and was as strong and vital as ever, and I would have trouble keeping up with him when he took a walk or did his martial arts movements. He would remain in this youthful state for six to ten months before needing to regenerate himself again.

These men and so many others have said the same thing regarding longevity: "Get chi and the rest will unfold and come." I have personally watched hundreds of vitality-filled older individuals prove this point.

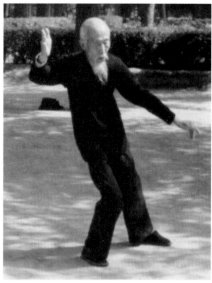

Liu Hung Chieh in his 80's practicing Wu style tai chi

Caroline Frantzis

Starting Tai Chi After Age Fifty

Clearly, the earlier in life you start practicing tai chi, the greater your physical and mental capacities will be in old age. However, like many people, you may ignore taking lifelong care of yourself until the natural vitality and regeneration abilities that you had in your youth start to wane. You begin to get wake-up calls. Suddenly that bump that used to heal in a day lingers for a week. Now when you stay up all night partying, sleep for an hour, and then go to work, you feel out of sorts for several days or a week. You may suffer from colds and other viral illnesses more often. Tension and anxiety seem to last longer. Your libido may decline. Your poor health habits are catching up with you.

Commonly, these wake-up calls happen to people in their fifties. Unfortunately more and more people are burning out younger and younger, experiencing these problems in their thirties and forties—some even in their twenties.

If you heed the wake-up calls, you will realize that you can reverse the damage and begin to regenerate yourself, regardless of your real age. Chronological age and functional age do not always go together. Tai chi's goal is to make you functionally younger.

Alternatively, you may be basically healthy in your fifties and recognize that keeping that health will mean you can continue to have an active working life, realizing the full potential of your dreams and making positive contributions to your family and society. When you retire, you can enjoy new adventures. Your goal may be truly to maintain, enhance, and heal, and you may begin looking for practices that will help you achieve this.

In China, half of the people who practice tai chi begin after age fifty. It was mind-blowing for me to watch so many older people regain the strength and vitality they had in their twenties and thirties. All practitioners talked about how doing tai chi made them feel better the whole day. Practitioners in their seventies and eighties told the same story, but with a much greater sense of gratitude.

It opened my eyes to the nature of living a whole life. As a youth growing up in the 1960s and 1970s I, like most every one else in my generation, believed life was basically over when you were old. And old was anyone over thirty!

Tai Chi's Special Benefits for Practitioners Over Fifty

Although all practitioners can expect to gain the health benefits outlined in Chapter 3, practicing tai chi has special benefits for people over fifty. Tai chi:

1. increases physical balance
2. regulates and lowers blood pressure
3. improves circulation
4. promotes a good night's sleep
5. re-establishes biomechanical alignments
6. restores sexual vitality.

Many health studies conducted in China show how tai chi and other Taoist practices improve health. Since the 1960s somewhere between one and two hundred million Chinese have done tai chi regularly to benefit their health. Their friends and relatives have seen and verified the results. There is a never-ending supply of positive anecdotal evidence regarding its efficacy.

Western academic studies are fewer and relatively new. In time, my hope is that studies will show tai chi's full range of benefits, including how it improves spine and joint problems, nerve dysfunction, postoperative recovery, physical rehabilitation from trauma (car accidents, falls, etc.), strokes, and sports injuries. Western studies showing how tai chi improves longevity are especially needed.

Physical Balance

For senior citizens, the fear of falling is a very real and serious matter. Poor balance commonly causes older people to fall and break bones, often resulting in unrelenting pain and difficulty for the remainder of their lives. Today, hip replacements are among the most frequently performed operations for the elderly. A study conducted by the United States National Institute of Health found that injuries from falls cost over $12 billion annually (and costs related to physical frailty were much higher[1]). For the aged, recovering from a broken hip can be a daunting if not impossible task.

Two Western studies sponsored by the NIH show how tai chi enhances balance and reduces the risk of falls.

A three-month study of 110 participants, average age eighty, conducted by the University of Connecticut, showed that tai chi helped produce a 25 to 50 percent improvement in balance.[2] A study of 200 participants over age seventy conducted at the Emory University School of Medicine, Atlanta, Georgia under the supervision of Dr. Steve Wolf and sponsored by the National Institute on Aging, found that tai chi resulted in a 47.5 percent decrease in injuries from falls. The study also showed a dramatic reduction in the participants' fear of falling: from 25 percent to 8 percent.[3]

The Emory Study suggested as the causes of improved balance the following attributes of tai chi:

- continuous movement
- small to large degrees of motion, depending upon the individual
- moving with flexed knees, with distinct weight shifts between the legs

[1] *Frailty and Injuries: Cooperative Studies of Intervention Techniques* was the name of an initiative undertaken by the National Institute of Health in 1990 to improve physical function in old age. The initiative helped sponsor studies at the Emory University School of Medicine and at the University of Connecticut's Health Center.
[2] L. Wolfson, R. Whipple, C. Derby, D.C. Judge, M. King, P. Amerman, J. Schmidt and D. Smyers. *Balance and strength training in older adults: intervention gains and Tai Chi maintenance. J Am Geriatric Soc* 44: 498–506, 1996.
[3] S.L. Wolf, H.X. Barhart, N.G. Kutner, E. McNeely, C. Coogler, T. Xu. *Reducing frailty and falls in older persons: an investigation of Tai Chi and computerised balance training. Atlanta FICSIT Group. Frailty and Injuries: Cooperative Studies of Intervention Techniques. J Am Geriatr Soc* 44: 489–497, 1996.

- the attention paid to developing a relaxed, upright posture, with the head and trunk straightened and extended naturally, with the sacrum not protruding backwards
- the rotation of the trunk and head as a unit during circular movements
- the eyes follow movement, promoting head and trunk rotation through eye centering and eye movements
- the asymmetrical and diagonal arm and leg movements of the form promote arm swing and rotation around the waist
- the constant shifting of balance and weight to and from each leg, building unilateral strength and balance, together with an awareness of one's balance limitations.

The Emory study suggested that the increased rates of falls in the other exercise modules studied simultaneously were due to the fact that these programs encouraged people to move quite fast.

The nature of tai chi helps people to appreciate the value of moderation—what I call the 70 percent rule (see p. 35). Giving 70 percent of your effort during practice, staying comfortable, and not over-reaching your capabilities, helps the body learn faster and pay attention to where imbalances may occur. In resistance or flexibility training there is a tendency to encourage people to go far too fast. That is when people get hurt.

Tai chi makes you more aware of how your body is moving in space, your physical relationship to objects and people in your environment. It also makes you better able to feel internal landmarks within your body such as your arms, spine, and hips, that tell you if your balance is solid or not. Although many exercises focus your awareness on your upper body, tai chi makes you equally aware of your lower body, which determines your balance. For many, age causes the body to lose its ability to feel, and with it goes physical balance. Tai chi increases your capacity to feel how your foot touches the floor and with what kind of pressure, which is essential to balance.

Tai chi also improves balance by:

- strengthening the leg muscles by continuously shifting weight completely from one leg to the other; lifting one foot off the ground while balancing on the other leg; and raising and lowering the body slightly in even, smooth, regular cadences
- strengthening the hip muscles by constant waist-turning movements
- straightening the spine, and thereby removing spinal obstructions which diminish the nerve flow that tells all your appropriate muscles how to react best to maintain your balance.

Lowering and Regulating Blood Pressure

A Western clinical study, done by the Johns Hopkins Medical Institution, showed that tai chi lowers blood pressure in seniors.[4] Sixty-two sedentary adults with moderately high systolic and diastolic blood pressure took part in the study. The study conclusively showed that tai chi's gentle movements were as effective in significantly lowering blood pressure as the higher intensity activity of aerobic exercise. It lowered systolic and diastolic blood pressure by 7.0 mm Hg and 2.4 mm Hg respectively over a 12-week period.

Tai chi uses a different exercise strategy for lowering blood pressure than the more common methods based on making the heart pump more strongly and faster, such as treadmill exercise or aerobics.

Tai chi lowers blood pressure by working with and directly stimulating your veins and arteries. By continuously alternating rhythmic pressures within your body, tai chi's movements create pumping actions that act directly on the blood vessels themselves. These internal pumps are built into the gentle rhythmic bending and straightening actions of the arms and legs that are part of every tai chi movement. These pumps regularize the blood pressure so it is even throughout the body, mitigating the tendency for blood to move slowly in one part of the body and fast in another. Tai chi's breathing techniques gently massage the heart muscle, which strengthens it and keeps it toned, just as regular massage does for ordinary muscles. Three mechanisms work together to create the heart massage: using the diaphragm, expanding and contracting the internal organs, and breathing from the back of the lungs rather than the front of the chest.

Because of this, tai chi can be safely done by those with severe heart conditions, where straining the heart is best avoided in general, especially in the postoperative recovery phase of surgery.

Improved Circulation

The effects of tai chi on the circulation of all fluids in the body are well known among its practitioners. Moreover, a study of 126 heart attack patients conducted showed that practicing tai chi exercises resulted in a reduction in diastolic blood pressure.[5] The authors also noted that most patients in the tai chi group completed the program.

Tai chi improves blood circulation through three basic means: intention, breath, and alignments.

---

[4] Deborah Rohm Young, Ph.D., Lawrence J. Appel, MD, MPH, Sun Ha Jee, Ph.D., and Edgar R. Miller III, MOD, Ph.D. *The effects of aerobic exercise and t'ai chi on blood pressure in older people: results of a randomized trial.* J Am Geriatric Soc 47: 277–84, 1999.

[5] K.S. Channer, D. Barrow, R. Barrow, M. Osborne, and G. Ives. *Changes in haemodynamic prarameters following tai chi chuan and aerobic exercise in patients recovering from acute myocardial infarction.* Postgrad Med J 72: 349–51, 1996.

1. **Intention**. Tai chi teaches you how to influence the movement of blood throughout the body by using your mind. It is based on two Chinese medical principles within the *Tai Chi Classics* (see p. 237), and built into tai chi's energy techniques: "the intention moves the chi" and "the chi-energy moves the blood."

2. **Breath**. Blood circulation often diminishes as people age, particularly the circulation to the hands, feet, internal organs, and spine. To bring blood to the hands or feet, simply focus your attention and breath into the more dead spots that you feel within them while performing tai chi's movements. This often results in the hands getting warm and the feet seeming to come alive. I remember training with Wang Shu Jin when he was in his seventies. He would teach tai chi outdoors during cold Taiwan winters and would hold out his ungloved hands to allow his students to get warmth from them. Over the years, Wang had stored a great deal of chi.

   The compressions and releases of tai chi's abdominal and diaphragmatic breathing powerfully moves blood within the abdominal cavity and lower back. This brings more blood to the internal organs and increases the blood circulation between them, both of which normally diminish with age. Specialized spinal breathing techniques and whole-back breathing moves all the muscles of the back, bringing blood to them.

3. **Alignment**. Proper alignment of the spine, combined with exceedingly gentle bending and stretching actions of the limbs, increases blood circulation to the entire spine and back muscles.

More Functional Biomechanical Alignments

Tai chi has an extensive science of establishing sophisticated body alignments that help chi-energy flow through the body (see Chapter 3, p. 55). This does several things to promote longevity:

- It relieves pain from your muscles and bones
- It prevents injuries by increasing your anatomical structural supports and improving your balance
- It heals joint and spinal injuries faster
- It strengthens the body for almost any kind of physical activity
- It improves the circulation of all bodily fluids.

Better Sleep

Elderly people often find it hard to get a good night's sleep. This is because many are fearful and stressed and their minds are metaphorically at war inside themselves. Insufficient peaceful rest during the night has two obvious negative effects; first, it makes people miserable and often hard for family, friends, and health care workers to deal with, and second, disturbed sleep wears out the nerves and the body. This causes people physical pain and general nervous agitation due to overt or subliminal emotional stimuli. This creates a vicious circle where imbalances in the energy of the internal organs can continue to agitate the mind. Conversely, unresolved tensions in the mind can unbalance the internal organs, creating pain and the symptoms of disease.

By practicing tai chi, the body, nerves, and mind become more peaceful, so it becomes progressively easier to get a good night's sleep—something which many tai chi practitioners are known to enjoy.

From the chi-energy perspective one of the primary reasons people can't sleep is that their energy gets stuck in their brain, which disturbs their acupuncture meridian flows. Tai chi helps to get excessive chi stuck in the head back down into the body through a technique call sinking the chi, or *chen* in Chinese (see p. 225). Consistent practice helps reprogram the body's tendency to keep chi in the head at bedtime and to stabilize it lower down at the appropriate times.

When all else has failed, you can try the following technique for dropping your chi naturally so you can sleep. While lying down, rotate both ankles one hundred times clockwise then one hundred times counter-clockwise.

Increased Flow of Chi

As you become progressively older, the more valuable cultivating chi becomes. If you just want its health benefits, you only need to do tai chi's external movements with some chi-energy content. However, for a long life filled with exceptional vitality and strength you should concentrate on integrating as much of the entire 16-part nei gung chi-energy cultivation system as possible into your form. It is integrating the Taoist nei gung system (which is explained in detail on p. 226), not just the sophisticated tai chi form movements alone, that regenerates the body and produces the maximum vitality and absence of disease over the long term. Metaphorically, the outer movements are the wine glass, while the chi methods are the quality of the wine inside. The outer tai chi form is a very systematic and effective vessel for simultaneously working all the benefits of chi deep into the body.

Tai Chi's Social Benefits

Tai chi provides one other essential component of longevity—it satisfies the need for social inter-action. As people get older, they may see their families and friends less and less frequently, isolating them from an important reason to stay alive—social interaction. For example, having a wife or significant other has been shown to extend the life span of men, although the case is not as clear for women. A growing number of seniors in the West are estranged from their families or live great distances from them. Few older people find that becoming personally alien-ated and socially isolated is conducive to a happy old age.

Tai chi classes help bring new relationships into our lives. With age it becomes more and more difficult to make interesting friends through normal social venues. Activities that provide powerful interactive situations where people can bond at a deep level are harder and harder to find. Tai chi classes are somewhat unique in that they put you in contact not only with members of your peer group, but also with people of all ages. Older practitioners often meet younger people with similar interests with whom they can share their accumulated life experience, skills, and wisdom.

Like golf, tai chi is a very mental activity. The sheer doing of it will keep you mentally active and alert. It provides a lifelong and very challenging learning experience. People often get as mentally stimulated reading and talking about tai chi as doing it. In this regard tai chi has a large volume of literature to be perused and Internet sites to chat on.

Tai chi classes provide one more necessary component for older people: human touch. Teachers use touch to correct the student's movements; students gently touch each other during two- and three-person practice exercises; the gentle forms of push hands also put people in direct contact with each other.

Tai chi has a long tradition of being done outdoors in nature. This gets you out of the house and reconnects you with the natural environment—a relationship that commonly brings natural peace and joy.

Better Sex From Youth to Old Age

Throughout the Far East tai chi is widely used to increase sexual appetite and pleasure. Millions recognize it as a reliable remedy for impotence, lack of desire, and the inability to function well, especially in old age.

Increased stress, tension, physical pain, and emotional imbalance all contribute to decreased sexual vitality. As you relax in body and mind, you increase the flow of chi and blood to every part of your body, including your erogenous zones and genital areas.

Tai chi improves sensitivity in the nerves in your whole body, especially your hands and mouth, so you can recognize and enhance pleasurable areas in yourself and your partner that could otherwise be numb or shut down. This enables you to feel and enjoy the nuances and rhythms of sexual excitement more strongly.

By strengthening and uniting the chi flow of the internal organs, tai chi increases your capacity to have better whole-body orgasms. Tai chi can teach you to pulse your whole body; for women this includes the vaginal muscles, which can heighten your partner's pleasure during lovemaking. Traditional Chinese medical doctors often prescribe acupuncture, herbs, and tai chi for restoring sexual vitality because they improve the energy of the kidneys, which, according to Chinese medical principles, is directly related to sexuality. These traditional methods carry far less risk of side effects than Western medications for impotence and other sexual problems.

Tai chi also helps in several other ways. It can internally massage the prostate gland, bring increased blood flow to the entire pelvic area, improve the flow of energy from the spine to the genitals, and make the hips and spine more flexible, mobile, and pain-free.

Tai chi increases the flow of chi-energy within both your body and mind. This upgrades the general level of your health, upon which sexuality rests. Chi-energy is the force of life itself. More chi equals more sexual vitality, and as your vitality improves, you feel sexier and functionally younger over time.

Light Weightlifting Training for Older People Using Traditional Weapons

Western research has confirmed that light weightlifting benefits older people both in terms of maintaining required muscle mass and preventing osteoporosis. Tai chi form training using weapons, especially heavier rather than lightweight weapons can realistically provide the same benefits.[6] For best results this form of resistance training is most commonly begun with the use of extra-heavy swords without sharpened edges, before moving on to poles and spears. For the truly fitness-oriented, extra-heavy broadswords with a maximum weight of between seven and ten pounds can be used until people are in their late seventies, but rarely beyond. (For more information on the use of weapons in tai chi, see pp. 131–35 in Chapter 7.)

---

[6] I cannot say for certain that tai chi practice reverses osteoporosis. During my time in China, I did not specifically look for or see clear cases of reversal, although I did see related benefits. Elderly practitioners constantly told me that tai chi definitely helped them in terms of speeding up the body's healing rate for broken or damaged bones, and related soft tissue problems.

All weapons training improves grip strength and physical balance, both especially important for the elderly.

Weapons training and tai chi may also give you stronger bones. When done with a stronger energetic (nei gung) flavor, tai chi is well known for increasing bone strength, called "creating tiger bones." Many tai chi masters in their seventies liked to demonstrate their tiger bones. They would ask young students to hand chop their masters' forearms as hard as they could. The students would yelp from the pain in their hands, while the masters would smile wryly or have a good laugh. When I was 16, my first tai chi teacher, Cheng Man Ching in New York City, played this hand-chop game with me, as did my next tai chi teacher, Wang Shu Jin in Taiwan, when I was 19. This created quite an impression as to tai chi's life-long possibilities!

Tai Chi for the Very Old

For the over-eighties, initial goals when learning tai chi are often very simple. You may only learn one or two movements a month, and although your movements for the first year may not be as well executed as those done by younger people, the benefits can be dramatic and life-affirming in the extreme.

Besides reducing or eliminating pain in all normal activities and reducing stress, practicing tai chi has many practical benefits for the very old. It can give you better balance, which will help reduce the fear of falling; improve leg strength to help you get in and out of chairs more easily; and provide the grip strength to securely hold a plate or cup. All of these abilities, which may seem trivial to a young person, make the difference much later in life between being functionally independent or feeling helpless.

Paul Shapiro

T.T. Liang in his seventies practicing Yang style tai chi

Conclusion

Tai chi can be especially beneficial in regenerating the vitality, stamina, and health for people over fifty. It is well named as "the longevity exercise."

T.T. Liang, top student of Yang style tai chi master Cheng Man Ching, began studying tai chi when he was around fifty. He became an accomplished teacher and attributed his ability to live to over one hundred to his practice of tai chi.

We are entering into an age where various forms of biotechnology offer the possibility of curing a wide range of previously untreatable diseases. Potential scientific advances could allow many to live twenty to thirty years beyond retirement. However, according to the findings of the science of gerontology, the most effective methods of achieving longevity will be low tech: exercise, good nutrition, managing stress, and getting a regular good night's sleep.

Growing old should be a pleasure, not just a struggle to survive increasing decrepitude. Mobility, balance, and a relaxed, peaceful demeanor will help you take care of yourself and make your family and friends able to enjoy and want to keep company with you.

Tai chi also increases functional independence, which can reduce the necessity of depending on retirement communities and nursing homes, or at least postpone this for some years.

Tai chi can challenge your creative energies and provide emotional and spiritual balance. It may enable you to discover new abilities and retrieve old ones. Tai chi is an engrossing activity that gets more, not less, interesting and fulfilling as the decades roll by.

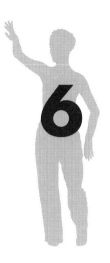

6 Tai Chi's Benefits for Different Groups of People

In China, the miraculous thing about tai chi is that different aspects of it appeal to different types of people, so that tai chi is ultimately able to appeal to and benefit all ages, all occupations, and all types of people in society. It is practiced by most to improve health, reduce stress, and aid longevity. Developing chi-energy is especially appealing to those interested in performing at exceptional physical and mental levels. Its martial arts aspects tend to appeal most to people under forty. Tai chi's spiritual practices take you closer to the profound—or at least help you to recognize your shortcomings with greater humility.

Tai Chi for the Young

A commonly asked question is "how young can a child begin tai chi?" The answer does not revolve around age, but the child's maturity. By age 14 or 15, most teens have the maturity, especially if classes are taught with a self-defense flavor. Children can begin earlier if they are not easily distracted and have the ability to be physically patient and methodical.

Most young children lack these qualities. They need to run, jump around, and make a lot of noise. In general, children and teenagers tend to be better suited to the more active martial arts of kung fu, karate, tae kwon do, or judo, rather than tai chi.

Tremendous physical education benefits, however,

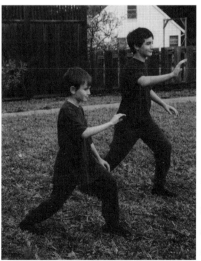

Caroline Frantzis

Children can begin tai chi once they have the maturity to stay still and keep focused without getting distracted do accrue when tai chi is started at an early age; benefits that normally are absent from formal and informal education from kindergarten through university. Through tai chi, youngsters learn experientially how to recognize the needs of the body and take care of it. This keeps them in good health and helps them attain optimum mental and physical performance.

Tai chi's educational process can help children in several ways. It can:

- increase their coordination
- provide them with practical skills to relax physical, emotional, or mental tension
- reduce negative buildup in their nerves
- achieve a sense of inner balance
- safely learn to develop flexibility.

Because many children bypass these simple, but important life skills, they can grow up living diminished lives. By turning off the desire for regular exercise, children get more involved in various forms of passive activities, such as playing computer games and watching videos.

Teenagers benefit from the process of learning tai chi thanks to its emphasis on patience, perseverance, and step-by-step development as a realistic and achievable road to long-term success. Through this they learn many valuable life skills. First, to recognize within their own body the boundaries of how much stress from work, study, or recreation they can handle, and, once this barrier is reached, how it must be realistically balanced with commensurate relaxation, thereby alleviating problems of excess and burnout.

Second, the innate quality of tai chi's slow movements graphically shows the young person how both success and failure build on each other over time. This not only shows the advantages and pitfalls of instant and delayed gratification, but it also gives a sense of time management—a strong indicator of success or failure in higher education or working life.

Tai Chi for People in their Late Teens, Twenties, and Early Thirties

Tai chi mitigates the effects of stress that many people begin experiencing in their twenties and thirties, which makes them age faster than their chronological years. For example, getting their bodies to relax deeply gives people internal emotional support. This can soften the massive hormonal swings that most youngsters in their teens and twenties experience. This emotional support helps people avoid negative behaviors to cope with stress, such as drugs, alcohol, and smoking. Tai chi can mitigate the damage of excessive life styles that many in these age groups engage in, helping people recuperate from "all nighters," and be able to sleep.

Because people at this age have abundant energy, they commonly do not realize that the tension they feel is cumulatively destructive. Tai chi helps them learn how to deal with stress and tension; as their bodies relax, their energy builds rather than dissipates. This gives them the added ability to "go for it" and attain high performance in any activity they choose with a great deal of joy. If, however, they continue to squander their energy, the tension will grow, their abilities diminish, and they will progressively weaken or damage their bodies and minds. When they hit mid-life or older, they may pay for these excesses in ways that can be quite unpleasant.

The Benefits of Tai Chi for People Who Work

There is something that many older students say to tai chi teachers. "I studied tai chi in college or in my twenties. It was wonderful in terms of how it made me feel and benefited my health. Yet I stopped. Why?"

Ten, twenty, thirty years later, the pressures of work, stress, and aging rekindle their interest because they remember how valuable tai chi was. At this point they commonly return and give it another go. Why? "I wanted to feel good again."

The largest component of the workforce comprises people between their late thirties and fifties. This mid-life period is classically the hardest period of most working lives. It is also often the most productive, as now you have both real experience and the energy to do something with it. During mid-life the pressure is on. Working, social, and family responsibilities rise year by year. If your health or strength weakens there are often younger people in line trying to get promoted over you, or take your job.

Tai chi gives you a much-needed competitive edge. It increases your capacity to withstand ever-increasing pressure gracefully. It boosts both physical and mental stamina, and helps you to relax more easily and recover from stress. More chi-energy increases your personal charisma and physical vibrancy, qualities that people want to see in leaders and co-workers at every level. It also generally keeps in check or lowers blood pressure that stress and poor diet aggravate with age, often to dangerous levels.

Tai chi benefits all sectors of the workforce in many ways. It increases productivity and creativity, whether you work inside or outside the home. It leaves you in better shape after the job is over so you can enjoy your time off, rather than merely recuperate.

Sedentary Office Workers

Prolonged sitting at a desk, with or without using computers, has associated occupational hazards which tai chi mitigates or completely resolves. These include the effects of poor posture, repetitive stress syndrome, and pain, especially in the back, neck, and shoulders. Utilizing tai chi will help improve productivity for the employer, and job security for the employee. Many tai chi techniques can be adapted to sitting in a chair (as practiced by the intellectual imperial elite in China for millennia), and short tai chi sequences or weight-shifting exercises (see p. 38 in Chapter 3) can be done intermittently during work hours—for example, while waiting for an important phone call or email reply, where you must either react quickly, or be in a relaxed mood to make a good impression.

Stress builds exponentially during the day. Taking time during coffee breaks or lunch to do tai chi can benefit you immensely. Simple tai chi routines can be done using only twenty or thirty square feet of space, such as a hallway. Many companies have outdoor spaces where tai chi can be practiced or in-house exercise facilities to reduce potential health problems and maintain the good health of their employees.

Carpal Tunnel Syndrome and Other Repetitive Stress Injuries (RSI)

Today's most common and growing RSI problem is amongst computer and other workers and is called carpal tunnel syndrome. The carpal tunnel is the space between the wrist bones and the ligament that holds the bones together. The median nerve is located there. The carpal tunnel space is naturally rigid, so if the soft tissues in the area swell, they compress the median nerve, resulting in hand pain and weakness. Repetitive movement of the wrists, such as prolonged typing or use of a computer mouse, can cause such swelling and lead to carpal tunnel syndrome.

Throughout the working world, chronic pain from RSI is a serious occupational problem. RSI can happen from working on computers, factory floors, or loading docks. It ruins many people's careers and their home lives too.

All repetitive stress arises when one or two anatomical spots take the full brunt, strain, and pressure of whatever action you continually repeat to get a job done. Tai chi physically and energetically helps prevent or cure this stress.

Causes of the Problem

Using computers requires you to bend your wrists and move your fingers to strike keys and move a mouse, often at similar bad angles, millions and millions of times.

Striking a computer key starts a tiny force wave that emanates from the point of origin, either in the fingers or wrist. This flowing wave will naturally move through and exit whatever is in its path, until it hits a bad angle where the wave is stopped and the impact lodges in a tiny specific, localized area. Usually the first stop is some point in the wrist for the fingers, or in the forearm or elbow for the wrist. At this point, the tiny force from your fingers transmits directly to that part of the arm, hitting like a lightweight hammer until every keystroke is painful. Over time this gentle but constant pounding strains and damages your wrist. After the wrist becomes habituated to hitting bad angles, a series of progressive strains and recurring pains happens within in the forearm, and then travels to the elbow, to the shoulders and shoulder blades, the neck muscles and vertebrae, etc.

These small pressures and strains on discrete pinpoint parts of the hand and wrist, etc., cause cumulative effects, just like single drops of water over time can dent and eventually wear holes through solid rock.

After your muscles tire, the ligaments and tendons take over until they progressively lose their spring and become fatigued. This destabilizes the fascia of your wrist. This in turn unravels the full function of relevant soft tissues and bones that connect to the next adjoining piece of soft tissue in your palm.

This binds and constricts the connective soft tissues and bones and they cumulatively begin to tighten. The blood vessels then become overloaded, tissues inflame and swell, nerve roots and carpal tunnel sheaths get irritated—resulting in dysfunction, the loss of finger and arm strength, and significant pain.

To prevent the problem, the forces with which you hit the keys or move the mouse *must not* concentrate only in one or two pinpoint parts of the fingers and wrist, etc. Rather they must be able to continuously transfer away from your wrist, to the next interconnected set of soft tissues, and the next, progressively up your arm, until the force waves diffuse and dissipate over larger and larger surface areas, such as your large upper back muscles, where there is minimal cumulative effect.

If the force wave gets stuck in a joint, tendon, or ligament, rather than passing through it, the force lodges there progressively causing damage, for as long as the spring in the soft tissues can handle it. When the soft tissues can't take any more, the force wave seeks each next new weak angle, one at a time, damaging them progressively in the same way. This process worsens the previous weak point as the force wave continues on the way to the next vulnerable spot.

When your muscles, tendons, or ligaments are not fatigued, but alive and springy, they can perform these micro-movements and effortlessly pass the force along to the next interconnected set of soft tissues. However, a bad angle of the fingers or hand position only gives you a tiny amount of soft tissue to generate the power to type or use a mouse, so the tissues fatigue easily. (Conversely by using your whole arm to dissipate small forces, you can repeatedly lift a three-ounce weight for hours with no problem.)

How Tai Chi Helps Prevent RSI

Tai chi helps prevent repetitive stress injuries in three ways.

1. Tai chi's movements create more micro-variation motions than normal in the specific places that affect carpal tunnel. It also conditions you to relax and let go of any kind of internal resistance you find anywhere in your body. By freezing soft tissues, these internal resistance points create the bad angles. However, even after fixing your current bad angles, new ones can emerge. Doing a tai chi form regularly fixes or lessens the new ones as they crop up. The form helps you subliminally learn which angles of impact will allow keyboard fingering or mouse actions to pass through any potential points of impact and dissipate

2. Tai chi movements constantly use a variety of different muscles so that various individual muscles don't get overused and fatigued.

   To accomplish any tai chi movement with fluidity requires you to continuously release all your bodily strength and tension without using muscular contractions. For this reason, the tai chi form demands you make ever-changing micro-movements inside your forearms, elbows, and shoulders. These constantly train you to smoothly re-sequence the flow of movement between all your different tiny ligaments and small muscles that are or could become frozen, thereby preventing fatigue to specific individual ones.

With practice, your awareness of your body and how it works grows, training you to re-sequence and relax your ligaments and muscles consciously. Over time these adjustments will become embedded in your unconscious reflexes. The soft tissues between the fingers and spine need to be sufficiently loose so they can move and continuously readjust to appropriate angles—freely, easily, and in an effortless, relaxed way

3. Tai chi improves the motion of the joints. Each one needs to have a complete range of motion in all angles the body is likely to use, so that joints can naturally and unconsciously readjust when needed. In many activities, joints are frozen in certain positions. If elbow or shoulder joints are frozen, pain will begin to accumulate there and create blocked micro-movements downstream in the wrists,

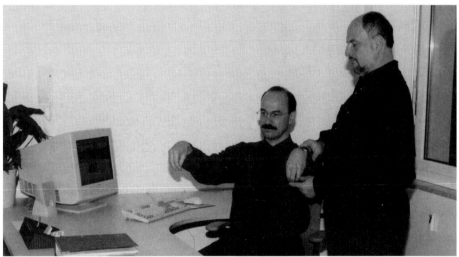

Tai chi movements can be adapted to help prevent RSI in computer users

palms, and fingers. These glitches block the transfer of force waves through the arms, thus generating bad angles.

Tai chi solves this problem with repeated, gentle rotations of the fingers, palms, wrists, elbows, and shoulders, as well as shoulder blade movements. These can restore the full range of motion to the joints and eliminate the possibility of forming bad angles.

Managers and Executives

Many executives and managers in Asia's tiger economies do tai chi to reduce stress and improve their personal productivity, thereby gaining competitive advantage. Tai chi's infinitely interesting and ever-changing puzzle keeps them on their toes.

Tai chi trains the mind to stay concentrated for long periods of time with a high degree of focused relaxation. These are essential qualities CEOs, executives, and managers need in any organization. Rather than giving you a specific intellectual technique, doing tai chi consistently trains your neurology, body supports (internal organs, etc.), and intent to get the most out of every moment, whatever the context. It does this in various ways:

- Tai chi increases physical stamina. It strengthens the energy that powers your internal organs, glands, and nerves, as well as reducing the stress work and life bring to bear on them. These factors, ultimately, are the source of physical stamina. Stamina is probably the single most defining characteristic of long-term success in all high-pressure executive environments

- It increases mental stamina. If your genetics have not given you incredible mental stamina, the mind's ability to concentrate must be exercised, nurtured, and grown, especially as you age. Tai chi is one way of doing this. Whether you are doing a form that takes one hour or one that takes five minutes, you should do the movements without physical stops and starts. Your whole being should be fully engaged, awake, and aware, never wavering or becoming distracted from whatever it is focusing upon during each specific movement. Ultimately this can only be done successfully if you become truly capable of relaxing your mind and increasing its ability to let go of anything extraneous to the task at hand. This helps train the mind to have the same relaxed, but alert, qualities while you are working. Significant mental relaxation increases mental stamina

- Tai chi increases mental flexibility. Being open-minded and capable of adapting to rapid change is crucial in today's executive offices. Doing tai chi movements places demands on you and brings out your hidden talents. Doing the movements constantly increases your level of physical flexibility while maintaining structural biomechanical requirements at the same time. To do both well simultaneously is mentally challenging and expanding. Doing both the external and internal movements well requires you to stay "on point" while being able to recognize everything that tangentially bears on the central point of each individual movement. This quality lies at the heart of efficiently organizing your own mind

- Tai chi increases calmness, awareness, and inner balance. Movements continuously alternate between left and right, up and down, forward and back, thereby causing you to mentally focus both internally and externally. Becoming more relaxed enables you to see many possibilities simultaneously, rather than only sequentially. This increase in awareness, coupled with the relaxing and calming down of your nervous system, enables you to see all sides of an issue and deal with the emotional undercurrents or explosions of others more easily. These skills are of benefit both for managers to get their teams to function efficiently, and for individual members within teams to collaborate well with each other
- Tai chi also helps your golf and tennis game, which can be an advantage in the world of corporate business and management. Its waist-turning actions can improve your golf drive, while the enhanced body sensitivity from either the form or push hands helps you to putt and volley at the net better.

Other Professionals

Many professionals work excessively long hours with heavy deadlines, and often do not get enough rest and sleep. A lack of rest diminishes productivity, which then requires putting in yet more hours to make up the deficit. Short tai chi breaks lasting a few minutes each during the day can relax your system sufficiently so that, in effect, you get sleep-like rest, and come back to your desk fully capable to engage in your work again.

How do short tai chi breaks manage this? By relaxing your nerves you begin to dump excess neurological overload that slows down your ability to be creative and manipulate or process information. Your nerve synapses can again function properly, allowing your nerves to recharge and your subconscious mind to regenerate. Emerging refreshed you can again assimilate and process information at your normal rate, and productively engage in the tasks at hand.

Clearing the charges or blockages that clog up your neurological system also creates a sense of internal space, an environment that often is the precursor for sudden problem-solving insights. This mechanism is like the common situation where you work hard on a vexing problem or idea all day and still can't figure it out. However, the next morning, after a good night's sleep has cleared some internal space, the solution seems to pop up out of nowhere. Artists and writers often use tai chi to get themselves in a creative mood, or to soften up their body and brain during the middle of a creative burst so that they can work longer before hitting a creative wall.

Tai chi stretches out the muscles of the neck, back, and shoulders too, preventing pain lodging in them. Nagging pain in these areas makes many prone to anger, frustration, and depression, which does not produce smooth working relationships. This pain also makes it harder to think, requires you to use a lot of disagreeable time squirming to get more comfortable, and reduces your productivity.

Tai chi also increases blood and energy circulation to and from the brain. When not enough blood gets to the brain you lack the "juice" to process information rapidly and make insightful decisions. Equally, when the blood does not drain from the brain the thought process becomes ponderous, as the brain seems to turn to mush and blood pressure rises.

Physical Laborers

If your work involves physical labor, tai chi makes your job easier and boosts your productivity in three ways.

1. It increases your physical flexibility so you can move better and faster, both in general, and more specifically to position your body more easily into those difficult-to-achieve angles that normally create physical strain.
2. When you are doing heavy lifting, tai chi educates your body to use its whole strength, especially the lifting power of your hips and legs, thereby creating less strain and allowing you to work more rapidly, efficiently, and with more stamina.
3. Tai chi creates looser, stronger, less tense muscles. This combination of increased flexibility and stamina prevents occupational injuries, especially those generated from bending, stooping, and squatting actions. This also helps prevent common back and shoulder injuries.

After work is over, doing tai chi reduces or completely melts away the physical strain and pain you acquired during your day. It helps to heal the small and large injuries acquired from work that do not initially require immediate medical care, but which often accumulate and progressively weaken the body. Unless taken care of, cumulative strains create the physical environment that can result in a major injury, like the proverbial straw that broke the camel's back.

Athletes, Dancers, Gymnasts, and Yoga Practitioners

Tai chi helps all athletes attain better performances—whether they are professionals, recreational athletes, or complete beginners. China's national sports teams regularly practice tai chi to improve their performance. As a subsidiary movement training program, tai chi upgrades the basic functioning of your nervous system, as well as your reflexes, flexibility, balance, coordination, speed, and whole-body power; both overall and for specific sports skills. The healing, stress-relieving, and meditative qualities of tai chi are especially appealing to dancers and gymnasts, who are more prone than most to frequent injuries to their muscles, joints, and spine.

The following list represents some of the special benefits tai chi provides yoga practitioners, dancers, and athletes:

- Tai chi can help prevent joint, muscle, and spinal injuries and thereby extend an athlete's peak performance years and prevent lifelong injuries or pain. Tai chi speeds up the normal healing time from injuries, so that less training time is missed. Tai chi's gentle motions bring more blood to injured areas, remove blocked energy, and help regenerate damaged soft tissues

- Tai chi gives athletes more perseverance and focus. To become really effective at tai chi or any martial art requires hard work, discipline, intelligence, and perseverance. Even practicing a tai chi short form promotes regular rhythms in an athlete's body and mind. This habit then makes it easier to keep up other rhythms related to basic conditioning and athletic skills both during and, more importantly, between competition seasons

- Tai chi increases speed, reflexes, power, and endurance, by increasing your reservoir of chi, upgrading, and making the central nervous system more efficient, and adding tone to the body's physical tissues. By subtly changing and supercharging your insides, you are able to manifest better external athletic performance abilities

- It improves left- and right-brain functions. This improves hand–eye coordination and general reflexes (especially useful for all ball and racquet sports). Practicing tai chi also increases the incidence of "time slowing down or seeming to stop," which high-level athletics seems to intermittently engender. Peripheral vision functions are improved too, so athletes can become more acutely aware of what is happening around them

- Tai chi relaxes and opens the joints and ligaments. This can stretch your arms and make them reach further, valuable for sports like basketball, and gives dancers more beautiful and fluid arm movements. Opening up the shoulder joint increases a pitcher's power
- The slow-motion movements of tai chi directly increase your clarity and calmness of mind, and help your central nervous system function more smoothly and efficiently. This improves timing and makes it easier and more common to achieve what in basketball is termed "being in the zone"
- Tai chi improves grip strength and sensitivity
- Tai chi reduces internal resistance and hesitation, so you can change tactics and strategies much more quickly. This also enhances your capability to instantly release explosive power
- Tai chi's emphasis on fluidly turning from the hips and waist improves power, balance, and fluidity of motion. This is especially useful for preventing joint injuries and enhancing the ability to turn suddenly from left to right—so critical when either generating power or faking opponents out in competitive sports like basketball, football, martial arts, or boxing
- It strongly develops whole-body coordination through an upper and lower body integration principle called the six combinations. This principle's objective is to make the whole physical body, chi, and mind move like one totally integrated cell or unit, with no parts moving separately. This is key to high performance sports and dance
- Precise body alignments prevent the flow of chi from being blocked or dissipated. This produces exceptionally effective biomechanical alignments, which can prevent injuries and allow you to use your body's full power
- Tai chi increases the speed and strength of the energy circulation in your legs, thereby bringing ease, adroitness, and spring into them. This improves general responsiveness, reflexes, lightness, and grace, and is equally valuable for long- and short-distance runners, dancers, gymnasts, and football players. It roots your energy to the ground, giving tremendous stability, balance, and maneuverability when skiing or lifting heavy weights
- Tai chi's methods of internal release, softening the muscles, and chi movement can show the yoga practitioner how to stretch farther without using muscular force or physical tension. Tai chi's energetic techniques, derived from the 16-part nei gung system (see p. 226), can make obvious what is hidden in Indian hatha yoga. This can be extremely valuable for inter-mediate and advanced yoga practitioners. See Appendix 3 for more on yoga and tai chi.

In terms of movement flow, tai chi has much in common with modern dance and induces a different kind of movement from most classical Western dance. In general, tai chi will relax the body more than dance or gymnastics. Many dancers, however, find that tai chi's slow motion movements do not satisfy their need to move in a more freeform manner. To gain the health benefits of tai chi through a different, faster approach, some dancers might want to investigate tai chi's chi-energy cousin, the internal martial art known as *ba gua* or *pakua*. Dancers usually find the greater speed of ba gua more satisfying. Many professional dancers over the years have commented to me that they find ba gua to be an amazing dance form, with its very unique movements, not found in other martial arts or the world of dance. Ba gua articulates every joint in the body in a multitude of circular and spiraling patterns. However, you must find a good teacher who understands the proper alignments of the hip, knee, and ankle joints, or else you might practice incorrectly and cause yourself knee problems.

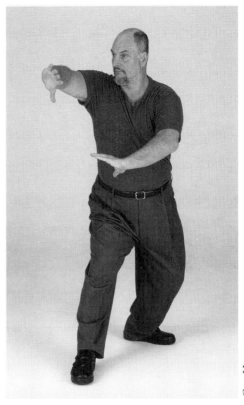

Guy Hearn

The author practices ba gua, a more dynamic internal martial art than tai chi. Ba gua is characterized by walking in a circle with frequent changes of direction. Unlike the slow–motion moves of tai chi, ba gua's twisting, spherical movements are usually done at normal or fast speed

Tai Chi for the Overweight

Tai chi is especially valuable for big people and those who are overweight because it is an extremely low-impact exercise. This issue becomes increasingly important the larger you are. High-impact exercise can cause damage to vulnerable joints such as the knees because of the weight impacting forcefully upon the joints and spine. Tai chi enables overweight people to handle their weight better and makes a difference to their day-to-day experience of health. Tai chi seeks to maintain, enhance, and heal the physical functions and strengths that make you healthy at any weight level, from extremely thin to very heavy.

To compensate for the potential health consequences directly related to excess weight, some degree of regular gentle exercise is even more necessary for the overweight than for the average person.

Tai chi helps mitigate the potential negative consequences of excess weight by building up your body:

- It improves your leg strength by having you constantly transfer your weight from one leg to the other. This improves balance and enables you to move better
- It improves your musculoskeletal system's ability to bear weight
- It improves the flexibility of your joints and spine. This reduces back pain and creates good posture
- It stretches your muscles out and improves their tone so that they are better able to bear your weight
- It improves your blood circulation, taking pressure off your heart.

Due to misplaced excessive zeal, overweight people often tend to overstrain the knees and back doing various kinds of exercise. In terms of tai chi the very overweight should bear in mind several points, including:

- the 70 percent rule (see p. 35), although if very unfit you may need to reduce it to 50 percent or less until your body significantly strengthens
- it is essential to maintain good biomechanical alignments for your ankles, knees, and spine. My book, *Opening the Energy Gates of Your Body*, shows some of these alignments for the knee and back
- don't be in a rush; you can only gauge how strong or weak your knees really are with patience
- only very, very gradually increase the degree your waist turns if you feel it causing even light strain to your knees
- do tai chi for at least six months or a year before attempting to do your form at a super-slow speed, such as taking an hour or more to do a long form (see Chapter 9, p. 179).

Tai chi emphasizes what you feel like, and how well your body functions, rather than your external appearance. Tai chi does not produce the "sexy" buff muscles seen on television exercise machine advertisements, nor any specific kind of body shape, such as the thin svelte bodies of fashion models. Whether being fat is socially good or not has a lot to do with fads, which change during different eras. It is extremely sad that young girls and women, thin in the extreme, literally starve themselves to death to avoid being what they consider fat and ugly.

Being fat is not a long-term health problem *per se*. Being weak and unfit is. If your added weight is diminishing your functionality, you can learn tai chi to make yourself stronger and you can create a positive self-image based on realistic health considerations.

Tai chi masters have been renowned for going into old age remaining very healthy and fit. For example, Wu Jien Chuan, cofounder of the Wu style, was a big man with a big belly. However, he was exceptionally strong and healthy well into old age.

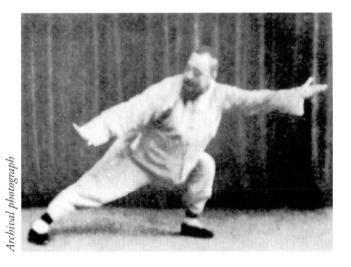

Archival photograph

Wu Jien Chuan, co-founder of the Wu style of tai chi. Despite being neither young nor slim at the time of this photograph, Wu shows his flexibility and strength by demonstrating a very low and extended tai chi posture

Tai Chi for People with Disabilities

Tai chi can be very beneficial for people with a wide range of physical and mental disabilities.

Hearing and Visually Impaired People

Tai chi helps both the blind and deaf develop better physical balance, which their handicaps often diminish. Lacking visual or auditory clues, they normally find it exceedingly difficult to compensate for physical obstacles in their environment. Both naturally develop a kind of sonar or radar to compensate for the lack of important visual and auditory clues around them. Through intensive energy work, tai chi masters were able to strongly sense what was behind them or function well with their eyes closed, as have masters of other martial arts based on developing chi-energy. The energetic skills contained within tai chi can strongly improve the radar and sonar abilities of the blind and deaf. The abilities can be gained though a combination of sensitizing the nervous system, slow motion movement, and working with the external aura or etheric body (see p. 60) and the meditative qualities embodied within the form.

People with Neurological Conditions

Even after normal intensive Western physical therapy, the neurological re-patterning and opening up of the acupuncture meridian channels tai chi offers is especially useful for improving the ability to move normally without spasms or distortions—problems that often follow polio, trauma, nerve degeneration from accidents, intense fevers, or diseases like multiple sclerosis. Taught by a talented instructor, tai chi can make the difference between being able to walk normally without the need of a cane and having a body that does not function properly.

Wheelchair Users

If you are wheelchair-bound but have the use of your arms, doing tai chi's arm movements will help keep the structures of the spine mobile and fluid. When you can stand, your physical therapy will most likely progress at a much greater rate and your recovery time may be dramatically speeded up.

Quadriplegics and paraplegics can also benefit from tai chi. By visualizing themselves doing tai chi, quadriplegics can often get their body's chi-energy and fluids moving better, mitigating the damage caused by total physical inactivity. It can also give them the impetus to internally straighten a collapsing spine.

Paraplegics can keep their upper body's energies flowing normally with tai chi's arm movements. Lack of leg movement pulls on the upper body's soft tissues, tightening them and diminishing blood circulation, both of which can create pain. Arm movements, combined with changing pressures inside the abdominal cavity can re-establish needed space between the internal organs, lift the spine, and stretch out all the tissues of the upper body sufficiently to alleviate pain.

Hand movements can work the energies within the legs through manipulating the external aura (see p. 60). This can significantly increase blood circulation in the legs, which can otherwise become diminished due to lack of movement. In this way, tai chi can reduce the damaging effects of leg atrophy on the whole body and brain. Sitting movements can also be focused to work and straighten the spine. In paraplegics, spinal vertebrae often collapse, causing negative cascading effects on the whole body.

For issues related to amputees and phantom pain, see p. 61.

People with Mental Problems

People with mental problems often live with brain dysfunctions that give them explosive frustrations and mood swings, which unhinge both themselves and others. Tai chi calms the nervous system, and helps release stress build-up, which can trigger the explosions. For these reasons, tai chi has been shown to be of value with post-traumatic stress disorder problems (see p. 87). Tai chi helps create stronger internal organs that can better withstand powerful emotional outbursts. For example, strengthening the kidneys may help depression to a limited degree, while strengthening the liver can reduce anger outbursts. Tai chi may also improve coordination between the left and right sides of the brain, which often helps people with mental problems.

Conclusion

Tai chi's ability to immensely improve the lives of people of many different ages and occupations is one of the reasons for its universal appeal. It can bring out and maximize the potentials inherent in most human beings, and diminish the damage that can occur from living a stressed-out life.

Tai chi is one of life's rare recreational activities that can become more interesting, challenging, and satisfying as life goes on.

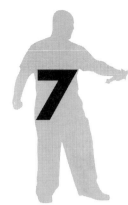

7 Tai Chi for Physical and Emotional Self-Defense

Chang I Chung, one of my first tai chi teachers, used to say, "Everyone wants to be healthy, only some want to know how to fight."

The martial arts celebrity Bruce Lee inspired millions of people to learn the hard style external martial arts, such as karate, kung fu, and kick boxing. Some learn a martial art as an insurance policy against being physically humiliated or abused, to physically protect themselves and their loved ones against violence, or to develop greater self-esteem and self-confidence. Others do it to fulfill their perceived warrior nature or for the sheer love of the art's sports-like aspect.

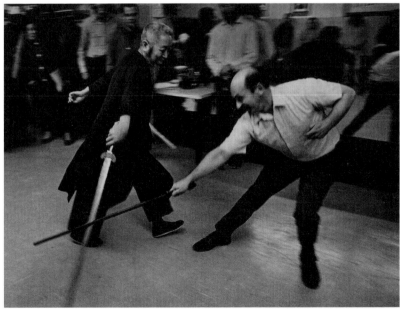

Ken Van Sickle

Yang style tai chi master, Cheng Man Ching, doing tai chi sword sparring with Lou Kleinsmith. Cheng was one of the seminal figures in American tai chi who emigrated from China and began teaching in New York City in the mid-1960's

Today, millions of people are actively involved in various martial arts; and tens of millions have at some time been engaged in learning karate, kung fu, kick boxing, etc. Although some teachers of all tai chi styles have a love and a bias toward teaching tai chi as an art of self-defense (its original purpose), such teachers of tai chi are significantly less available in the West than for the "hard" martial arts mentioned earlier. Since the 1990s, however, the public has been inspired and intrigued by the ideas of chi-energy portrayed by the entertainment industry's ever-present versions of the martial arts, such as the TV program *Kung Fu*, the movie *Crouching Tiger, Hidden Dragon*, and Japanese anime cartoon shows like *Dragon Ball Z*.

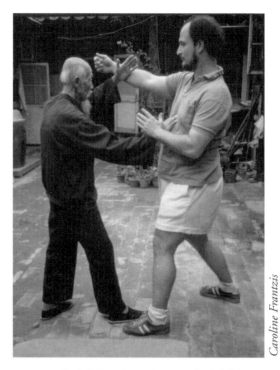

Caroline Frantzis

Liu Hung Chieh deflects the author's punch and delivers a finger strike to the solar plexus using the beginning of the tai chi move Fan Through the Back

Tai chi is one of the few genuine and accessible sources where anyone can find out how chi-energy really works. What gives tai chi its special power and speed to be an effective fighting art, from youth through to old age, is the infusion of the chi-energy principles that have been used for millennia primarily to improve health and longevity.

How Tai Chi's Slow Movements Create Fast Fighting

Many people are frankly skeptical that tai chi is a martial art. They ask, "How can anyone defend themselves in slow motion?" This is a reasonable question if you have only seen tai chi done in slow motion.

However, the perception is inaccurate, as tai chi does have training methods that allow practitioners to move at exceptionally fast fighting speeds. Here are five examples of how practicing tai chi's slow movements translate into the ability to fight exceptionally fast:

1. Tai chi tones and relaxes the muscles. The more relaxed and toned muscles are, the faster they can move
2. Tai chi trains the central nervous system to be more efficient. The nerves then give strong signals to the muscles to move faster
3. Slow-motion movement acts like a kind of weight on the muscles, which, when removed, causes them to move faster.

   Try this experiment to understand this idea experientially.

   Have someone time your quickest speed for moving your hand from the side of your hip to the top of your head. Then do the same movement in extremely slow motion. Now relax as much as possible, and go *really slowly*, for example taking five minutes to move your hand from your hip to your head and another five to come back down. Next try the same move at full speed, and see if you can move faster than your previous quickest time. It is likely that the more you relax when you move slowly, the faster you can go when you try to move quickly
4. Tai chi gets your whole body movement coordinated. Efficiently linking your waist and legs can really help catapult your hand speed
5. In more advanced practices, you learn to seamlessly alternate between doing extremely slow and fast movements, first during solo forms, then push hands, and finally during sparring. Your chi controls your nerves and muscles like an electric light's dimmer switch, which can gradate light from almost total darkness (excruciatingly slow motion) to extreme brightness (lightning fast).

Tai Chi as an Effective Martial Art

In the nineteenth century, tai chi proved itself to be an exceptionally effective, practical fighting art. Tai chi teaches the timing, fighting strategies, and presence of mind necessary to succeed in unrehearsed fighting with someone who has aggressive lethal intent and cannot be psychologically dissuaded. Until the 1920s, the martial side of tai chi was normally emphasized. However, sometime during the 1930s, tai chi began to be taught purely from the perspective of health and longevity. From that time forward, many teachers downplayed or completely eliminated its use as a fighting art.

Today, only a small minority of practitioners are sufficiently skilled in using tai chi's martial arts techniques to effectively teach how to counteract the most severe of violent circumstances. However, there are some teachers who can show a few of the fighting applications either with or without making martial arts the main focus of the class. Nevertheless, the overwhelming majority of tai chi teachers and practitioners do not know the martial arts aspects, and therefore you cannot expect them to teach you tai chi as a practical fighting art.

The Difference Between Internal and External Martial Arts

Although all forms of martial arts are advertised as being effective for fighting and self-defense, few specify whether they are external or internal martial arts. Consequently, many people don't understand the term "internal martial arts." Is the martial part something like karate where people grimace, shout, and break bricks? Does internal mean that unlike other martial arts, you don't punch, kick, chop, throw, or use arm locks to defend yourself against aggression in dangerous situations? Does internal mean practitioners can point their hands at someone twenty feet away and mysteriously kill their attackers, send them flying through the air, or at the least knock them down without touching them? These and other misconceptions abound.

All martial arts were originally developed for mortal combat and have arsenals of fighting techniques specific to their styles. The difference between internal and external martial arts is in how they train practitioners to acquire their speed and power. External martial movements look, feel, and are different from internal martial art movements. *Internal* refers to how internal martial arts invisibly get their physical power, not what their specific fighting movements look like. Internal movements are most effective if they are imbued with the knowledge of how chi-energy can be specifically incorporated into fighting techniques, which shows you how to make the movements come alive and be effective in combat.

Internal chi-energy techniques can make the muscles relaxed, strong, sensitive, fast, and extremely responsive.

Internal martial movements can look as though something invisible within the practitioner is moving their body. The more a tai chi practice is coming from an internal aspect, the more the relaxation and fluidity shows in their body movements. True internal movements also appear to have great hidden energy and a sense of tangible presence that doesn't waver.

The source of the power of tai chi and other internal martial arts, that mysterious *chi*, comes from developing the energetic components of the 16-part nei gung system (see Chapter 11, p. 226). You can do the same movement in an external or internal way, but the differences lie in exactly how you use your mind, body, and energy to make the movement happen. For example, with an external technique, keeping your elbow in a certain specific place develops physical habits that either deny your opponent an opening or leave you wide open and defenseless. Internal techniques deal with whether and in what way the elements of the 16-part nei gung system are being implemented.

In general, external martial arts depend on external movements and tend to use more linear fighting techniques. Internal martial arts use both visible external movements and invisible internal movements and emphasize circular fighting techniques. Internal power methods rely on developing chi-energy rather than the external muscular tension and strength, for example, that you would gain by lifting weights or doing push-ups.

The external martial arts, such as kung fu, boxing, jujitsu, karate, kenpo, kick boxing, and tae kwon do, generate powerful movements from tense, stiff muscles and use muscular strength, bursts of physical tension, growls, and sometimes overt aggression that is often catalyzed by the release of adrenaline. External movements have a sense of hardness, force, or strain behind them. Internal movements are soft and effortless and seem to the opponent to come out of nowhere. However, an internal martial artist's movement can have at least as much or more strength and power as the same movement from an external martial artist.

At the highest levels, predominantly external martial arts include some soft, circular, or internal techniques. Other external martial arts, however, may have many internal techniques woven through their external methods. Such martial arts are called internal/external if these internal chi methods are significantly more prevalent. An internal martial art such as tai chi, however, does not include external practices and uses purely internal techniques. For example, using these criteria, in Japan, aikido would be classified as an internal martial art; ninjitsu as an internal/external martial art; and karate as an external martial art.

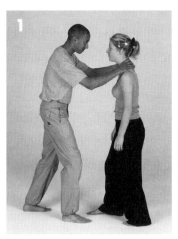

*Escaping from a choke
and counter-attacking
using the tai chi movement,
White Crane Spreads
its Wings*

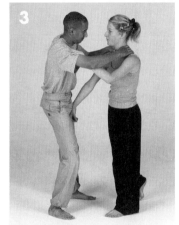

1 Opponent attempts a choke

*2 Turning the waist to escape
from the choke and positioning
the lower hand for a counter-
strike*

*3 Pulling the opponent off-
balance while doing a groin
strike—a classic snake move*

*4 Positioning for a strike to the
head by keeping the opponent
off-balance and bringing the
lower hand upward between
the opponent's arms*

*5 Finger strike to the oppo-
nent's eyes with back foot
poised to kick*

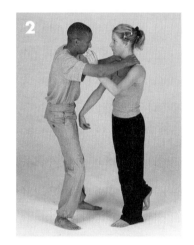

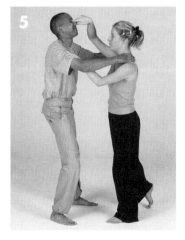

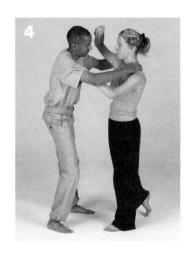

The internal martial arts, for example tai chi chuan, hsing-i chuan, ba gua chang, and aiki-do, generate movements from chi-energy. Practitioners' bodies move in a relaxed, soft, and fluid manner. The internal martial arts do not encourage overt emotional aggression and anger as a primary power source. It would be difficult for a layman to comprehend how tai chi's slow movements can translate into fast fighting. The uninitiated would be even more baffled by the concept that fighting methods that do not engage emotional aggression and anger can be as or more effective than those that do.

Seven Stages of Learning Tai Chi as a Martial Art

For tai chi to be functional as a martial art, you must know how to use its fighting applications when facing a real person. Otherwise, during solo practice, your visualizations about how to apply the techniques will be false and will be unlikely to translate to the real thing.

Tai chi taught for health and longevity does not normally provide the detail and practice needed to apply tai chi in a combat or self-defense situation; tai chi taught as an effective fighting art will. During solo practice, you are taught how to focus your mind to defend or attack. You are taught when to mentally pause or unleash; how and where to hit, at what angle; and what kind of intent and internal power to use. You are also taught multiple fighting applications for each and every movement within a tai chi form, what specific kinds of chi allow them to work, and how and where to use them. (See *The Power of Internal Martial Arts*, Chapter 4.)

For the layman, one way to describe learning tai chi as a martial art is in seven basic stages that are like a circle. With each succeeding revolution, you accrue greater skill as you revisit and upgrade the same material in greater and more satisfying depth.

The seven stages are learned both empty-handed and using traditional weapons such as swords, poles, and spears. The process is as follows:

1. Chi-energy warm ups, which eventually include the entire 16-part nei gung
2. Solo form, with several aims:
    a) to obtain the physical coordination required to move well with relaxed power

b) to learn punches, kicks, joint locks, throws, etc., specifically related to each
form movement

c) to develop chi power, so that when you hit or throw someone it counts

d) to develop the internal strength to withstand punishment without caving in

3. Self-defense practices with a cooperative opponent. This begins the process of
understanding how a real person feels and responds. At first, techniques are done
at slow speeds with minimal power, until you can stay relaxed without tensing up
and not rely on external, muscular power. Then you learn and practice how each
individual technique within the forms can be modified to be equally effective at
long, medium, or short distance. This level of training may either be done concurrently as you learn the form, or immediately afterwards. Tai chi schools without a
true self-defense orientation usually skip this stage, even if they include push hands

4. Push hands is an important bridge between doing the solo form for health and
learning the realities of fluid self-defense with dangerous determined opponents.
An essential stepping-stone in self-defense, push hands shows you how to bring
invisible internal power, to be used later in sparring, into your body movements.

During push hands you maintain constant touch with your partner's arms. Using
all the chi-energy techniques hidden within the tai chi form, you attempt to push
your partner without being pushed yourself. The subtle internal power skills
learned during this stage will be the same ones that you will execute when making contact with an opponent who is determined to cause you grievous bodily
harm or death. However, to be an effective tai chi fighter, push hands alone is
not enough. You must also progress through the next three stages

5. Sparring games. One or more people attack you, demanding that you apply the
basic self-defense methods of tai chi in various attack–defense scenarios. These
may be done in choreographed sets or spontaneously. Like boxing, tai chi techniques are begun in close, then at arms' length, and then yet farther away. To
begin with you will know what is coming and at what level of speed and power.
Progressively, your opponent will attack with more intense speed and power, and
varied footwork, encouraging you to better adapt and be more effective in your
defense. Later, attacks and defenses get more fluid and devious with yet more
power and speed. Eventually you will be limited to using specific tai chi techniques, but your attacker will not be. Now the timing and mind games begin,

upon which real fighting revolves

6. Next comes the true transition between push hands and fighting. Here you apply the internal power skills you learned in push hands to hit, kick, and throw, as well as to push your opponent while still maintaining continuous physical contact

7. Unrehearsed sparring is the final stage. It is only at this stage that you learn to use tai chi's full range of fighting techniques to deal with both known and unpredictable variables.

Practicing with Traditional Chinese Weapons

Before firearms were introduced in China, traditional weapons such as swords, poles, and spears were used both for military warfare and self-protection against criminals, civic unrest, and general lawlessness. During the nineteenth century, martial artists from the Chen Village, the birthplace of tai chi, were trained to use a wide variety of arcane weapons, such as iron fans and three section staffs. This was just as vital a part of their training as learning empty hand tai chi forms. Today, however, virtually all teachers of tai chi as a martial art instruct in only the use of four weapons: the straight double-edged sword, the broadsword (sometimes called the saber or big knife), the pole, and the spear. Although firearms have rendered them obsolete for fighting, learning to use these weapons has many benefits in terms of developing your body and chi, either for health or martial arts. They are normally introduced in tai chi training only after empty-handed tai chi forms are learned.

For health, an important goal of weapons training is to solidly project chi from your body through and to the end of each particular weapon. The more you can do this, the stronger and more connected the chi-energy inside your body will become. Physically, the use of these weapons progressively develops different parts of your body in the specific order given below, so that learning a new weapon both continues and increases the previous benefit and adds something new.

For martial arts training, learning to use weapons increases the speed of your hand and foot movements and amplifies the power to your arms and hands when you practice empty-handed forms. Weapons training also familiarizes you with moving more to back and side angles in different ways than in push hands or empty hand forms. Most sparring is like push hands with implements, with the techniques of sticking with and anticipating your opponent's force emphasized just as much. For safety, use weapons with blunt, not sharp edges or points, during solo and sparring practice.

Straight Double-Edged Sword

The swords are commonly made of wood or steel. Extra-heavy steel weapons are often used in solo training only, rather than real combat, and ideally weigh between three and seven pounds.

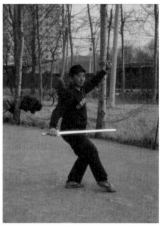

Caroline Frantzis

Head instructor at the Beijing City Physical Culture Institute in 1986, demonstrating the Yang style tai chi sword form with a double-edged straight sword

Health   Generally considered the most elegant and beautiful weapon, the straight sword's trademark is finesse. It builds wrist flexibility, whole-body movement, and increases the fluidity and sensitivity of your arm joints. It also is an excellent training device for enabling the waist and legs to connect to the upper body and hands in a finely coordinated manner.

Martial Arts   The straight sword is the first and most commonly taught tai chi weapon. It emphasizes stabbing and cutting actions and finesse over raw power. It is better for fighting one-on-one duels rather than multiple opponents. In ancient China, the straight sword was the fighting weapon of choice for female martial artists. It emphasizes the basic technique of cutting the inside of the opponent's wrist to disarm or fatally bleed him or her. Being double–edged it trains the ability to rapidly and sensitively change from twisting inwards to outwards—a critically important capacity in tai chi's empty hand fighting applications and push hands.

Sparring   Trains complex footwork patterns and deliberately develops softness and fluidity in hand and foot movements in order to attack or defend from unusual angles. Using the sword helps you to give up the bad habit, at least for tai chi, of using muscular force while fighting. The tai chi classics talk about the sword being so sensitive that a fly cannot land on it without setting it in motion. To use brute force with a weapon that sensitive will most likely result in you getting cut first. The traditional weapon was extremely sharp and strong, and was perfect for techniques that take almost no power, in order to attack and cut veins, arteries, and other especially weak and vulnerable vital points located only a few inches inside the body. As such, straight swords do not require the power to hack and completely split the body wide open to be fatal.

Broadsword

Broadswords are commonly made of wood and steel. They are straighter on the bottom and curved on the top. Extra-heavy steel weapons are often used in training only, rather than real combat, and ideally weigh between four and ten pounds.

Health Broadsword solo practice develops physical strength and flexibility, especially in the wrists, shoulders, neck, chest, and upper back. Although a power weapon, it adds flexibility to the shoulder blades, neck, and chest through movements that bring the sword around your neck and back before returning it in front of the body to cut.

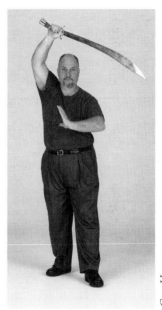

Guy Hearn

A tai chi broadsword movement used to deflect a blow to the head from another weapon

Martial Arts Primarily a man's rather than a woman's weapon, the use of the broadsword emphasizes power. Many techniques are geared toward hacking off limbs, decapitation, or cutting completely through the torso. Its strong point is fighting multiple rather than single opponents. In contrast to the straight sword it develops power more than sensitivity, uses large sweeping motions rather than small tight ones, and emphasizes stabbing actions much less than the straight sword. Many of the body positions and techniques are not unlike those used when fighting with Japanese samurai swords.

One side of the sword is thick and strong rather than sharp. It enables you to absorb especially powerful blows and then immediately counter–attack with the sharp edge. Broadsword fighting includes more athletic moves like jumping kicks, stomps, and spinning techniques uncommon in tai chi's straight sword or empty hand methods. Currently, the broadsword is not taught very much in the West, although this may change in the future.

Sparring   Broadsword sparring methods only partially emphasize a push hands-like scenario, where two broadswords stick together and maintain continuous contact.

Poles

Poles are traditionally made of wood, and are between six and nine feet long, reasonably thick, and of equal circumference throughout. Ideally the wood itself is either very heavy or flexible.

Health   Provides resistance training, and it is especially beneficial for increasing the strength and flexibility of the entire back and spine.

Martial Arts   Provides superlative additional training for tai chi's twisting and spiraling techniques (see pp. 216–21). An omni-directional weapon, it focuses on bringing power instantaneously to any point along the entire length of the pole. The weapon adds many new defensive perspectives for dealing with opponents either to your back or side. A primary goal of the pole is to maintain control of the weapon. Ideally, even if the weapon is powerfully hit, you don't take any shock into your body, and can immediately counter. Its primary techniques are to poke, stab, smash, and be able to bring sharp, snapping, vibrating, or penetrating power to either end of the pole.

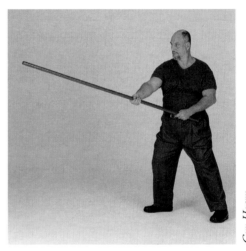

Guy Hearn

A parry and attack with a pole. Tai chi pole techniques emphasize the ability to stick to, and thereby control, the opponent's weapon

Spears

The spear is known as the king of weapons in China because no other non-projectile weapon can defeat it. The classic spear is between seven and nine feet in length, with the bottom being slightly thicker than the top. Normally the spear's head stabs, while its sides cut.

Health   Especially works the leg muscles and opens up the chi power of the legs and lower tantien. Of all the weapons, the spear offers the greatest potential to extend the body's chi externally.

Martial Arts Develops tremendous body maneuverability, and combines the techniques of the pole and straight sword within its fighting repertoire. Its basic technique involves a powerful twisting parry culminating in a powerful forward stabbing or cutting motion, often combined with a strong vibrating action.

Both the pole and the spear are used to develop the ability to discharge energy, called *fa jin* in Chinese. See Chapter 11, p. 236. They do so by creating vibrations within the lower tantien, shaking the weapon's tip, and creating very strong twisting within the practitioner's entire body and weapon. Both techniques train you to instantaneously bring power into empty hands or weapons especially from the difficult beginning position, with your hands being lower than your hips.

Canes and Sticks

Today it is not practical to walk the streets with any of the four weapons just described. However, a cane or walking stick can easily be adapted to many of the basic techniques of the four traditional weapons to devastating effect for self-defense. Some tai chi schools have developed walking-stick forms for this purpose. Only a little creativity is required to make the conversion.

A tai chi overhead strike using a cane

Michael McKee

Push Hands

Many tai chi teachers will bring in some form of gentle, non-threatening push hands into their classes because it is an effective tool for training relaxation. Relatively few teachers, however, know how to specifically use push hands as a realistic self-defense training tool. Push hands eventually can become as intense and rough as any contact sports.

In push hands, you and your partner's hands or arms touch and ideally remain in contact during the entire exercise through three basic progressive stages.

1. The weight of both practice-partners alternately shifts completely from the front to the back leg. Partners usually move forwards during attack and backwards during defense

2. Both partners continuously turn their hips and waist from the front to the side, in coordination with attack and defense moves. This is the first step in unifying the power of the whole body for maximum physical efficiency

3. As both partners move back and forth, their hands, forearms, elbows, shoulders, and possibly even hips engage in gentle or very serious attack and defense flows. Ideally all movements are much more circular than linear.

Neither partner tries to hit or kick the other, only to unbalance and push. Only in the most martially orientated push hands styles, like the Chen, is it permissible to also throw or apply joint-locks. All push hands is done standing up, albeit at times in a very deep crouch. No wrestling on the ground, pins, strangles, or other mat work techniques are involved.

The goal is not to use overt muscular strength to overcome your partner. Rather it is to rely on relaxation, intent, awareness, sensitivity, and moving chi-energy through your body to produce the subtle yet significant physical power necessary either to withstand an opponent's onslaught, or to project power from your body to push or uproot your opponent.

The basic circular push hands strategy is "one half of the circle defends, and the second half attacks." For defense, the focus is on grounding (rooting), deflecting, or yielding, rather than opposing the opponent's force. But, a split second later, the goal is to counter by returning your opponent's force back to him or her, by unbalancing or pushing rather than hitting or throwing as in jujitsu or karate.

Push Hands Helps Manual Laborers
Prevent Repetitive Stress Injuries (RSI)

The practice of push hands trains practical skills of whole-body power that can prevent RSI for manual laborers. It educates you to use progressively more and more of your whole body's power to do a task that needs strength, rather than only using a single part of the body, such as a shoulder, wrist, elbow, or lower back to take the brunt of a task, which over time results in chronic pain and loss of function. (See also Chapter 6, pp. 108–112.)

The focal point of repetitive strain is in the incessant use of backs, shoulders, knees, elbows, and wrists, which over time can result in chronic pain. In the case of manual workers, tens or even hundreds of pounds of force are applied when workers lift, rotate, push, bend, or stoop to manipulate different tools, work industrial machines, or move objects around. The result may be constant pain and lack of functional strength in areas that can cripple you.

Push hands teaches very sophisticated ways to either absorb or send force out of your body with minimal repetitive stress to vulnerable body parts:

- Push hands awakens and trains all the small muscles needed to transfer force waves through specific areas of the body so they continue to function properly. In this way, heavy pressure doesn't repeatedly land on a specific place—a shoulder, for example—slowly but surely weakening and damaging it

- In its rooting training, you learn to transfer weight from its origination point smoothly through all your body parts, until it dissipates into the ground without straining your body. Even if muscle strain occurs, it is evenly distributed throughout the whole body and not localized in specific joints or the spine and lower back. This is done through proper biomechanical alignments that allow you to bear weight dramatically better and reduce the chances of industrial accidents

- Either to stop someone's force from entering your body, or to send your full body's power at your practice partner, you constantly turn and rotate your joints. This prevents your whole body's force from getting blocked within them. This increases the ability of your joints to avoid getting hit by repetitive cumulative strains when either absorbing (bearing weight) or putting out force (moving something)

- The process of learning to issue internal force shows the body how to lift or move heavy objects without damaging individual body parts, especially the back, knees, elbows, wrists, and spine. Maintaining proper biomechanical alignments and other techniques allows force to travel efficiently and smoothly from your feet, through your legs, up your back, and out of your arms and fingers.

Fixed and Moving Push Hands

Both partners are immensely challenged and enjoined to never break physical contact during the two basic methods of doing push hands: fixed and moving.

In *fixed push hands*, the feet remained fixed on the ground and do not move. As both partners continuously shift weight back and forth, each does a repetitive fixed pattern of specific arm movements. These incorporate the four major energies of tai chi: up, back, down, and forward, called in Chinese *peng* (ward off), *lu* (roll back or absorb), *an* (press downward), and *ji* (press forward). Later, over time, your arm and waist movements are no longer fixed within a specific form and both partners are encouraged to spontaneously respond according to the tactical needs that arise moment by moment.

In *moving push hands*, the feet move using progressively more complex patterns.

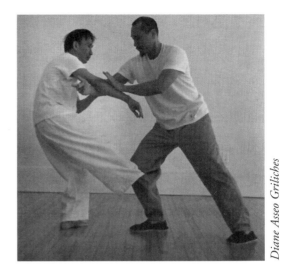

Instructors practicing Moving Push Hands *at Brookline Tai Chi in Boston*

1. Using the same fixed hand patterns previously learned in fixed push hands, you add fixed repetitive dance-like steps: moving forward, to the back and sides, in zigzag lines, or in semicircles

2. Maintaining the same unvarying footwork, your hands are allowed to spontaneously move anywhere your intuition and judgment lead

3. Both hands and feet move spontaneously

4. You now add a different set of fixed hand and foot patterns, called *da lu* in Chinese. This focuses on difficult diagonal angles of movement, especially 45-, 135-, 225-, and 315-degree angles

5. Staying within a very loose adherence of *da lu's* attack and defense methods your feet and hands become relatively free-form

6. Free-form push hands now encourages you to freely mix and match at will all tai chi's hand and footwork moves from both fixed and moving push hands. Both partners are now free to push hands spontaneously in any way they like.

In time all the principles of fixed and moving push hands are applied to traditional weapons, mostly using straight swords and poles. Push hands is also a powerful tool for reducing stress and for emotional defense.

Diane Asseo Griliches

Is Tai Chi the Best Martial Art for Self-Defense?

Like Formula One car races, it is ultimately the driver, not the car, which determines victory. If we use the baseline of those with similar natural talent, dedication, and the willingness to put in the necessary "whatever it takes" effort and time in their training, some basic comments can be made.

In the short term—less than a year or two—external martial arts give a more reliable minimum level of self-defense competence than tai chi. Long term—with a time horizon of ten years and more—the balance shifts to a more internal direction. This can be seen in many Japanese and Korean martial arts where at the higher black belt levels, circular, soft, and internal techniques are often considered the choicest meats of advanced training.

Although many martial arts schools advertise "instant self-defense," these claims are often very exciting but ultimately based on hype. Most middle-class people have not fought on the streets all their lives. They are not psychologically or physically used to responding to extreme physical aggression without freaking out or becoming paralyzed with fear. In reality, and with the best of training, assuming no firearms are used, it will take quite a while before a middle-class person can expect to walk through a really nasty neighborhood with any reasonable confidence of surviving a physically violent confrontation.

Two things are necessary for successfully using self-defense skills: psychological attitude and effective physical technique. Both hard physical linear technique and external strength go online faster than the soft circular techniques and internal strength tai chi employs.

Many external martial artists don't think tai chi works. Even after they see a tai chi person "kick someone's butt" they don't believe it, for several basic reasons.

First, tai chi is not a psychologically aggressive martial art. Most humans are conditioned to the idea of fighting by our biological heritage. Animals growl, become tense, and noisily violent, either in order to dominate a weaker

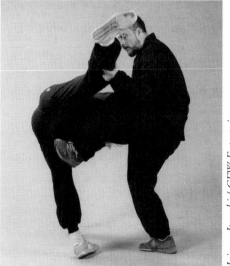

Jaimee Itagaki / CFW Enterprises

Using the tai chi movement called Deflect, Step Forward, Parry and Punch *to deflect an opponent's kick and break his leg* animal, or fight off a predator. Tai chi takes the opposite approach. It trains you to be emotionally calm during combat—relaxed, psychologically neutral, silent, yet exceedingly physically effective. This is harder to achieve and takes longer than the biological animal approach.

If a tai chi practitioner vanquishes someone, the opponent usually won't be given any emotional cue of dominance. It appears as if the victory was by accident, rather than a deliberate act. Consequently, a Doubting Thomas won't really believe his eyes, because of the absence of visible facial expressions and emotional verification.

Secondly, because tai chi's internal power is invisible, you have to feel it to believe it, not see it. Not all tai chi masters feel compelled to demonstrate their power or cause people pain to prove something. And some martial artists can't believe it's not all a pretense unless you cause significant pain. So the choice may be to hurt your opponent or be considered a fake.

Third, some metaphorically expect a tai chi master to walk on water, when it may only be possible to be a strong swimmer. Not everyone is at the almost supernatural levels of skill that are portrayed in movies. In this sense, the situation is comparable to the mythology often seen in movies surrounding karate black belts who are supposed to be able to kill with one blow. In fact, few can achieve this, and many, if not most, cannot even reliably do one-punch knockouts, especially against opponents with hard heads.

Finally, it takes years to become reliably good, with finely honed techniques that consistently work against people who can fight well. Only a minority of tai chi practitioners knows its basic arsenal of kicks, punches, throws, chokes, etc., much less its full range of fighting techniques. Because of tai chi's emphasis on psychological relaxation and non-reactive emotions, to reach this level usually takes five to ten years, practicing for several hours four or five days a week.

However, if you are not in a rush, you can learn tai chi self-defense skills that may one day stand you in good stead, while acquiring the potential health, healing, longevity, and spiritual benefits for which 99 percent of practitioners take up tai chi.

Do You Have to Learn Self-Defense to get the Health Benefits of Tai Chi?

The simple answer to this is no.

However, knowing some simple fighting or self-defense applications for each move will help you remember some of tai chi's choreography and how to string the moves together in longer and longer sequences. Simple fighting applications help you remember how to move chi from point A to point B in your body, both within each move and in the transitions between them. It is difficult for anyone not trained in movement and dance arts to remember long sequences of relatively complex movements, much less the even more complex energetic movements. The traditional and effective way the more qualified teachers were trained was by showing how specific postures would be used for self-defense.

Your intent moves your chi. Thinking of either hitting or deflecting physical attacks with hands or feet automatically activates your intent, thereby moving your chi-energy to the desired location, provided that you have learned the necessary specific details. At first, most people have trouble remembering and then visualizing all the movements and technical energetic details. Self-defense metaphors are more easily remembered than most other memory techniques.

For those who abhor anything that smacks of violence, it is worth considering that if you have no violence in your heart, internal visualizations (mental pictures) of self-defense moves do not create the future seeds of violent intent. Rather, they only become schematics for moving chi and thereby benefiting your health and spiritual wellbeing.

Emotional Self-Defense

Emotions, at their appropriate times and in balanced proportions, make life smoother and more enjoyable. However, when your emotional balance is greatly disturbed you may involuntarily hurt yourself and others, either physically or emotionally.

Tai chi generally, and push hands specifically, physically and psychologically help balance your emotions by smoothing out the excessive secretions from your internal organs that make you pre-disposed to certain damaging emotions, described in Appendix 2.

The Taoist philosophical principles of tai chi are very real and accessible to the trainee. These pieces of ancient wisdom carry over into the psychological arena and give you excellent tools to soften the potential emotional shocks and blows of life. These work well on many levels for a stressed-out world.[1]

Excessive aggression often can make you uncontrollably angry. Anger can cause you to say and do things impulsively that you may later regret, with an offendingly stressful level of force many don't appreciate. Because you can't emotionally slow down and understand what is

---

[1] For more information, see *The Power of Internal Martial Arts* (North Atlantic Books, 1998), pp. 290–92.

going on, you may not look before you leap. The stressful emotional havoc that anger can wreak on yourself or others, either through lost friendships, unsatisfying relationships, creating enemies, or the need of others to get even, is physically and emotionally debilitating. The emotionally softening tai chi principles of "following and yielding to an opponent's force" can help circumvent the endless emotionally painful situations that fill the lives of many.

Emotional bullying is common. Without being obvious, this same yielding to force principle can enable you to psychologically refuse an emotional bully a solid place to hit, control, or coerce you into doing something to which you fundamentally object. Another tai chi quality, "strength within softness," makes many bullies lose interest in using emotional force on you, as they intuitively know it will not be worth the trouble. "Listening to and interpreting your opponent's force or energy" trains the emotionally unperceptive (those who are constantly putting their foot in it), to become more sensitive and aware. This quality also makes people more predisposed toward useful co-operation rather than needlessly stressful confrontation.

People who are not emotionally grounded often can't make decisions, as they fear making mistakes or making others unhappy. For others, being assertive and standing up for themselves is extremely difficult. Both conditions often make people feel their lives are emotionally out of control—a less than joyous situation for most. Psychologically implementing the tai chi principle of "being rooted without being stiff" can be of great help in finding a strong emotional center, and can be very liberating.

Tai Chi's Value for External Martial Arts Practitioners

If you are adept in an external martial art, such as kung fu or karate, tai chi and other internal arts will help you increase your arsenal of fighting techniques. More importantly, they will help you learn how to apply chi-energy to the movements you already know, and thereby expand your martial creativity. Tai chi can also give interesting insights into your external techniques and make them become alive and new again. And it is, of course, valuable and enlivening to exchange martial arts information with students of internal styles.

Tai Chi's Value for Older Martial Artists

In America and Europe, millions of people have practiced and enjoyed external martial arts for a year or two when younger, but then have had to stop due to the pressures of work, school, or family life. When they are older, some of these people feel that they might like to begin again. However the more external martial arts—karate, judo, tae kwon do, or boxing—are mostly a young person's game, for many reasons:

- They are hard on the joints and spine.
- Training injuries are part and parcel of external martial arts training. However, as you age, the body heals more slowly.
- The young are psychologically more likely to be attracted to violence than older people.
- The young have natural energy to burn, which diminishes as they get older.
- As you age, you are likely to feel more pain from training the same amount of time, and ache more and longer afterwards.

Older martial artists want something they can actively continue into old age that their body can handle and which will reduce rather than increase the stresses in their life.[2] They want a martial art that will calm them down, rather than feed their aggressive tendencies. Tai chi is a natural fit, and currently many karate and kung fu schools are adding tai chi to their curricula.

It is extremely common for top-level external martial arts masters and senior practitioners in China, and even in Japan, to take up tai chi after they pass the age of fifty. At that age few are trying to become high-level tai chi specialists. However, these martial artists recognize that doing a tai chi form is a practical way to extend their physical skills many years past the point at which these abilities would naturally decline in their own martial art. This is because tai chi can make them healthier, heal old injuries from decades of training, make the body less brittle and more flexible, and maintain the speed of practitioners' movements.

In the West there are many older martial artists who have been practicing for ten, twenty or thirty years and want to continue. After the age of fifty, tension slows them down more than it did when they were younger and makes their practice time hurt more. Lack of minimum speed eventually takes the fun out of doing most martial arts for older practitioners. Tai chi keeps the hips oiled and moving with speed and power, which lies at the heart of virtually all martial arts. Many, especially those between forty and sixty, find that tai chi enables them to speed up the

---

[2] See *The Power of Internal Martial Arts*, pp. 286–89.

techniques they normally do, so that they can perform them even faster than when they were young—or at a minimum, not get any slower.

For seniors with decades of martial arts experience, learning tai chi from a master who knows its self-defense tradition thoroughly usually gives new and fascinating martial insights. When an old dog learns new tricks it usually makes him feel happy and young again.

Conclusion

Tai chi was first developed as an effective martial art that incorporated internal principles of chi development known to the Taoists for thousands of years. Counterintuitively, its slow movements can develop the extremely fast responses and movements that fighting demands. Tai chi instills the ability to fight in a relaxed, soft, and focused manner, without the anger and aggression that is often characteristic of the external martial arts, such as kung fu and karate. However, today relatively few teachers teach it as a martial art, although some may teach a few fighting applications to help students remember the moves.

8 Tai Chi and Spirituality

Tai chi is an art, not a religion. To practice tai chi you do not have to believe in gods, spirits, the tao, or an afterlife. There are large numbers of tai chi practitioners of all religions. Yet many consider the practice of tai chi to be a spiritual practice. There are several reasons for this. The line between *art* and *spirituality* is often very thin. Techniques of art can stimulate creative forces and refine them. If that intensity is directed toward inner discovery, rather than external accomplishment, the training that the art provides may bridge the gap between the secular and the spiritual. If so, art thereby becomes a tool for spiritual awakening. This can be the case with the practice of tai chi.

Tai chi contains within it much of the East's philosophy and wisdom that is immensely practi-

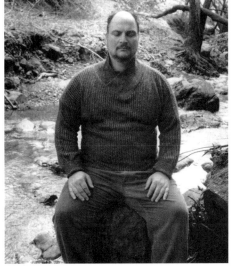

Craig Barnes

The most internal aspect of Taoist tai chi's moving and sitting practices deal with learning how to free the spirit. It is here that the full potential of tai chi as a form of meditation can be realized

cal and useful for our daily lives. This includes the wisdom it applies toward health and relaxation; to chi-energy in the human body and mind; and to strategies for dealing effectively with the practical matters of business, conflict, and human relationships. However, except in a few legends, tai chi does not claim to be divinely-inspired. It is the wisdom of men and women seeking to make this earthly life work well. Yet, the line between wisdom and spirituality can also be blurred, as wisdom is often gained through various spiritual practices. For all these reasons, the philosophy underlying tai chi is often taken to be spiritual.

Tai chi chuan was developed as a martial art, drawing heavily upon ancient philosophical concepts shared by many Chinese systems of thought, including Taoism, Confucianism, some schools of Buddhism, and traditional Chinese medicine. Although the energy work of tai chi originated with Taoist monks, I know of no evidence that indicates that tai chi was developed for spiritual or religious purposes after it emerged from the Chen village and was spread by the Yang family. (For more details on the styles and spread of tai chi, see Chapter 9.) I had informal conversations about this subject with the tai chi master Yang Shou Jung after he accepted me as a student. He was the great-grandson of Yang Lu Chan, who founded the Yang style of tai chi. When I asked if he taught meditation, he said that this was not, and had never been, an aspect of his family's training, which was about chi development and martial arts.

How Tai Chi Touches on Spirituality

Today, the word "spiritual" is used to describe a multitude of experiences without a defined common thread. Let's look at some common perceptions that people use to describe spirituality and how they specifically relate to secular tai chi.

- **Spirituality allows you to make contact with or become something larger than your individual self.**
  From this perspective tai chi is spiritual. The feeling emerges when a normally disconnected body and mind connects. The sense of internal unity this generates is definitely larger than your normal sense of "me." Athletes temporarily experience this feeling when they are "in the zone." Regular tai chi practitioners commonly find themselves in a "larger than me" sense of time suspension where past, present, and future merge into a fourth kind of timeless dimension. Many describe this as a personal, intimate contact with an indefinable and satisfying spiritual quality
- **Spirituality is something that gives an appreciation of the divine or God, whether through words of scripture or experiences of nature.**
  In my opinion, no writings within the field of tai chi are intended to rise to the level of words of scripture. Although some phrases within the tai chi classics are taken directly from Taoist spiritual texts, taken as a whole the *Tai Chi Classics* do not approach the level of a divine work (See Chapter 11, p. 237, on the *Tai Chi Classics*).

However, tai chi can engender an appreciation of the divine through an experience of nature. Tai chi is often done outdoors and gives many a direct spiritual connection to nature that is above and beyond that normally obtained from simply physically being in a natural setting. Some describe this as an experience with the strength equivalent to the sense of divine presence felt in prayer. As said in an earlier chapter, "If you take one step towards God (the divine), God (the divine) takes two steps toward you"

- **Spirituality means having a regular practice.**
For many people, commitment and regularity are essential aspects of any coherent philosophy of life that is geared toward awakening spirituality within. Regularity of practice allows one to go beyond intermittent outward shows of spirituality.

    Tai chi's solo practice regularly produces an internal rhythm within its practitioners that is the equivalent of a spiritual metronome. This rhythm helps you focus on the more subtle, indefinable spiritual qualities of life. This focus is activated within the extremely truthful situation of being alone: here all you will find is what is inside you, whether spiritual or not. This inner solitude is where direct, personal communication with the divine is consistently known to happen, in all spiritual traditions

- **Spirituality is often associated with a return to a lifestyle in accord with the divine or natural moral "spiritual" laws of the universe.**
Spiritual inquiry is often framed within the ancient debate of how to achieve virtue through morality. This may be done through activities of a more outer or inner nature, such as:

    a) taking actions or thinking thoughts that are supposed to be pleasing in the eyes of God (the more Western view). Tai chi does not address this subject. In some tai chi schools you may find practitioners discussing how tai chi might relate to these issues, but such discussions are generally based on their own personal religious beliefs, and not something inherent in the practice of tai chi

    b) following and understanding how the laws of karma work (the more Eastern view). You try to engage in the world in a manner so that your actions and thoughts benefit rather than harm yourself, those you care about, or those you don't personally know, now and in future lives. In Christianity, the concept of karma is echoed in the biblical phrase, "as you sow, so shall you reap." Although tai chi does not discuss karma openly, its principles of soft and hard, empty and full, absorbing and discharging by extension work with karmic laws

c) engaging in a profound study of ethics, to raise us to our highest or spiritual possibility. In China most tai chi people follow what is called martial arts ethics: *wu de* in Chinese. The central issue of *wu de* (and the whole of tai chi) is achieving balance—not only inside the body, but within the rough waters of maintaining good and honorable human relationships, now and into the future.

- **Spirituality is often associated with practices that enable people to feel more coherent and open inside.**
  Tai chi can achieve this, especially as practice becomes more regular. Doing the form regularly has a way of creating internal cohesion and openness. This happens in other spiritual practices using other methods, such as prayer, visualizations, mantras, yoga, sitting meditation, or performing sacred dances.

In the inner traditions of the world's major religions, spirituality involves the process of exploring, finding, and remaining in a divine or spiritually open state all the time—often referred to as "enlightenment," with all that entails. In Eastern traditions, the capacity to concentrate deeply is one major essential ingredient needed to become enlightened. In this regard tai chi helps you develop various extremely subtle concentration abilities.

Will the Practice of Tai Chi Conflict with my Religion?

Tai chi is not a religion. Tai chi is about awareness not beliefs. Its spiritual side neither affirms nor denies the existence of any specific god, gods, spirits, or an afterlife. As such it doesn't conflict with other religious beliefs.

If you specifically learn and practice tai chi as a Taoist moving meditation method, this will help increase your awareness of the human condition, and help you delve into your inner being or soul. You will not have to change your religious beliefs. However, indirectly it may cause you to appreciate some normally ignored aspects of these beliefs.

The practice of tai chi may make you feel more spiritual. Those spiritual feelings can be interpreted and directed within the belief system of your own religion. When one of my Catholic students was asked whether tai chi conflicted with his religion, he said, "I am a Roman Catholic and I believe in God. I believe that God created my body and the energy to use it. Tai chi helps me to appreciate my body and to access and use this energy effectively. Therefore, on the level of nature, tai chi helps me to better understand and enjoy the wonder of creation."

Meditative Movement: Secular Tai Chi

Tai chi is commonly called moving meditation. This phrase is derived from the Chinese, *dong jing*, where *dong* means to move, and *jing* means to be still, which is a classic term in Taoism for the English word meditation.

The common meaning of the term in English, however, does not imply all that is meant in Taoist meditation. Moving meditation in English merely implies that tai chi's movements are done in a meditative way, which is how 99 percent of commonly found tai chi is done. For this reason, we will call such meditative movement "secular tai chi," to distinguish it from the purely spiritual context of Taoist meditation. Secular tai chi means to maintain a relaxed focus, quiet one's internal conversations, and do movements in slow motion with a deep sense of relaxation.

The secular meditative movement aspect of tai chi is, however, only a shadow of the full implication of the deepest spiritual levels of Taoist moving meditation. There it connotes a deep inner stillness that can stably and permanently live at the heart of one's spiritual being. Inner stillness is a central goal of both Buddhist and Taoist meditation methods. From the classical Eastern perspective, meditation goes far beyond popular Western conceptions of spirituality as discussed above. The full opening of your inner being (or soul), or enlightenment, is meditation's central focus. This opening allows your heart and mind to become truly free. It is a subject to be learned by deeply exploring your inner landscape over many years, using extremely sophisticated practices and techniques honed by practitioners over hundreds of generations.

Secular Tai Chi Can Build a Foundation for Meditation

Many people who are interested in meditation are slightly afraid of it. Without knowing why, they correctly sense they may encounter inner conditions that they have spent their life avoiding and denying. I once asked my late Taoist meditation master Liu Hung Chieh why he didn't teach Taoist meditation to more people. His short and succinct answer was "Not many want to learn."

Secular tai chi may provide a useful buffer zone, allowing some to bridge the gap and eventually engage fully in deeper spiritual exploration. It is an excellent way to build the kind of foundations all forms of meditation or deep levels of spirituality

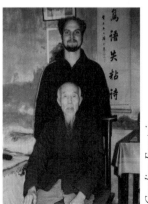

Caroline Frantzis

Formal disciple portrait of the author and his Taoist Lineage Master, Liu Hung Chieh

initially require. These include:

- constancy of purpose
- the ability to go within
- the capacity to recognize and apply progressively more subtle levels of your awareness
- focusing for extended periods on specific inner qualities with minimal distraction
- being relaxed, without which the previous requirements are going to be difficult to sustain.

Secular Tai Chi Can Help Meditators of Any Spiritual Tradition

Secular tai chi can be practiced by meditators of all spiritual and religious persuasions as a body-oriented practice that is complementary to the core practices of their meditative traditions. If you are primarily involved in mental or intellectual practices, tai chi helps keep your body healthy.

Many religious and meditative traditions are essentially intellectual practices. Everything takes place in the head. These practices primarily involve:

- auditory techniques, using prayer, mantras, repeating the names or words of divine beings, etc
- visualizations of deities, angels, spirits, saints, heavens or hells, or of various natural or esoteric realms, etc
- third eye meditations, many of which focus on the psychic planes, with practitioners observing mentally either energy or the mind moving through various spheres of existence, including their own body.

Often meditators cannot process or balance out all the mental and psychic energy unleashed within, which causes the mental energy these practices generate to become stagnant and unintegrated within their physical body. This is especially true for those with sedentary lifestyles. If meditation and religious practices are not complemented with some way of working with the body, this can create immense stress. The potential result is that the brain can suck excessive energy out of the body, making the practitioner devitalized, weak, and often sick. This situation exists equally in the East and the West, in meditation traditions both conventional and esoteric.

An ever-weakening body can create obstacles to progress in meditation. When sufficiently weakened, energy does not smoothly flow through the body's energy channels. This creates different kinds of body noise due to the irregular energy flow through the nervous system. People then confuse body noise with internal mental phenomena; the very obstacles their meditation is supposed to transcend, and which cause the meditator to chase down false internal leads *ad infinitum*, and waste practice time.

Meditation traditions rarely recognize this need to prevent potential health problems. However, a few traditions do, and incorporate some physical exercise. Such traditions include:

- Hatha and some other forms of Indian yoga
- Tibetan Buddhism, which adds some yoga practices, as taught in some of the schools in the West
- twirling or dancing in some Sufi schools
- Taoism, where all its meditation schools incorporate some body practices, such as chi gung.

Endless mental or psychological examination alone won't make your body function at anywhere near optimum levels. Intellectual brilliance doesn't ensure physical prowess. Many famous saints have been known to end their days with broken, pain-racked bodies.

Those Western meditation schools that do encourage body practices generally recommend such Western exercise such as aerobics, weightlifting, running, etc. Often the only specific physical practice Eastern schools use within the context of meditation is taking short walks, for example in Buddhism's Vipassana and Zen schools. This alone, however, is rarely enough to keep the body in good condition.

Secular tai chi, which emphasizes both balancing internal energy channels and building health, can provide a needed balance to intellectual and meditative pursuits.

Taoist Moving Meditation: Taoist Tai Chi

For thousands of years, most genuine schools of Taoist meditation have used chi gung exercises to develop health and wellness, and provide the bridge to Taoist moving meditation practices. The internal methods of tai chi were adapted from millennia-old schools of Taoist chi gung, which used entirely different movements (see p. 15). Commonly, longer chi gung sets had as many or more physical movements as tai chi and were done only for health or spirituality.

During the nineteenth and twentieth centuries, some Taoist meditation schools adapted the spiritual techniques within long chi gung sets into tai chi forms. For the purposes of this book, we will call such tai chi "Taoist tai chi" or "tai chi as Taoist moving meditation."

In the Taoist tradition, the road to spirituality involves more than having health, calmness, and a restful mind. The goal of Taoist meditation is to directly connect with your soul and free the deepest recesses of your being, and the highest purpose of meditation is to make you aware of the permanent, unchanging center of your being, that place of spirit and emptiness that is Consciousness itself. This level is beyond mere physical and mental relaxation; rather, it is relaxing into your soul, or your very being. (The Taoist meditation tradition is explained in detail in my books, *Relaxing Into Your Being* and *The Great Stillness*.)

To commit to this path is very much like going to a religious school for many years. In this tradition, spirituality does not come like a bolt from the sky, just because you want it. It is a subject to be learned by deeply exploring your inner landscape over decades.

Once you have health and peace of mind, you are ready to embark on three key stages towards achieving the goals of Taoist meditation. Only after you have more or less fully completed one stage, are you ready to embark on to the next. The three stages consist of the following:

1. Becoming a fully mature human being who is wholly free of inner conflicts and inner demons. Taoist meditation helps you completely release all the small and large conditionings, tensions, and blockages that bind and prevent your soul from reaching its full spiritual potential
2. Reaching inner stillness. Taoist meditation brings about a place deep inside you that is absolutely permanent and stable. It does not waiver, whether you are quietly sitting or are involved in doing fifty things at once
3. Transforming the body, mind, and spirit through internal alchemy.

The stages of Taoist meditation can only be taught by a living Taoist master and, depending on the school, may be taught as sitting, standing, moving, or sexual practices. As with any tradition, within Taoism there are many schools and subdivisions.

Exploring Non-Duality: Understanding the Underlying Nature of Opposites

Many of Taoism's meditation practices seek to allow you to penetrate, negotiate, and transcend the underlying nature of opposites. In order to transcend opposites you must come to understand and fully experience the principle of non-duality. According to the non-duality principle, there is a state or place where all seeming opposite yin-yang qualities (night–day, high–low, good–evil, male–female, etc.) originate, exist, are the same, and can cease. Any yin-yang pair at a deeper level implies several possibilities. Is it this (yang)? Is it that (yin)? Is it neither this nor that? Is it both this and that?[1]

In Chinese this state of non-duality is called *tai chi*. This philosophical concept is implicit in, and a natural extension of, the Chinese philosophical principle of *liang yi* or *yin-yang* (see Chapter 1). Here, simple or complex potential conflicts or disturbances that can arise between any set of yin and yang opposites can be resolved.

In English, the specific terms used for many of these yin-yang resolutions are found in the *Tai Chi Classics* and sound very strange and off-putting to the average Westerner. For example:

- form is emptiness, emptiness is form
- from stillness comes movement and from movement comes stillness
- to open is to close and to close is to open
- seek the straight from the curved.

In secular tai chi, these yin-yang principles are explored in the context of your body. In moving meditation and Taoist tai chi they extend into all realms of human experiences, from the emotional and mental to the psychic and spiritual.

In the Taoist meditation tradition, three presuppositions pervade all these yin-yang, non-dual principles, which cumulatively are parts of what is called the "road to (inner) maturity" and "inner stillness."

1. Whatever is within the deeper recesses in your psyche is not set in stone. So if something is tearing you apart inside, it is possible to release all your internal conversations about the perceived hurts, all the resentments, all the "they made me do it," or "they did it to me," etc. You can release all the internal limitations your past has imposed upon you, and through which you create your self-identity,

---

[1] These four possibilities in Taoist philosophy are called "the four corners" and are implicit in any yin-yang relationship. They are also central to the Madhyamika or "middle way" philosophy, which, according to the Dalai Lama, underlies Tibetan Buddhism.

which now dictates how you should act and think. Your past does not have to be your future.

2. Meditation gives you the power to truly take responsibility for your life. This is not necessarily for how external events will turn out, but most definitely for your interpretations and responses to the trials and tribulations life throws up. This frees your spirit from unnecessary internal burdens as you travel the road to becoming internally free.

3. Most people think, "I am my personality." Taoism holds that you are truly something more than your personality.

The Taoist Tai Chi Tradition

As noted above, there exists a rare tradition of people who use tai chi to achieve the goals of Taoist moving meditation. They interweave within tai chi's physical movements specific energetic techniques to help achieve the three stages of Taoist meditation (maturity, inner stillness, and alchemy).

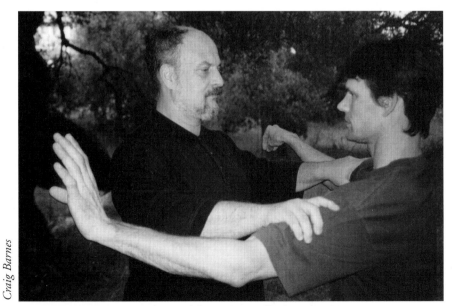

Craig Barnes

Meditative attention is required when learning tai chi for spirituality

Many of the martial arts masters I met in China were aware of the tradition, but few knew tai chi masters who had transformed the practice of tai chi to a complete Taoist moving meditation method. Such meditation and tai chi masters shared this tradition only with practitioners who had achieved a high degree of proficiency in the energetic aspects of secular tai chi (but not necessarily its martial aspects) and had a sincere desire to embark on a spiritual path.

The religious sage and tai chi master, Liu Hung Chieh, my last teacher in China, was one of those people. I was very fortunate to be accepted as his disciple in Taoist meditation and, specifically, tai chi as a practice for achieving the goals of Taoist meditation.

Today there are few recognizable schools of Taoist tai chi in the West. Very few masters know Taoist tai chi and are willing to teach it. Usually those who claim to do so are mainly teaching tai chi as a meditative movement to achieve health and calmness. They are teaching secular tai chi, not Taoist moving meditation or Taoist tai chi.

Only after you have achieved health and calmness, and know and can do the movements of tai chi with minimal effort, can you study tai chi as a spiritual method of achieving the goals of Taoist meditation. This is not something that you can do by yourself: you need a Taoist tai chi meditation master.

Achieving Maturity

The first stage of Taoist meditation is to become a fully mature human being. Mature individuals can relax and function well amid life's imperfections, without the need to be acknowledged for their accomplishments or to pass judgment on others. Through the maturity practices, you move towards a personal freedom from conditioned emotions and thought patterns, which may take years of practice. As long as you possess internal demons that obsess or depress you, you cannot become internally relaxed and natural. To become mature, your innermost soul must relax and free itself of these conditionings.

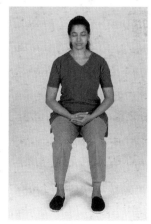

Guy Hearn

Taoist meditation can be done seated comfortably in a chair. You do not have to sit on the floor cross-legged or in a lotus position

Finding Inner Stillness

The second stage of Taoist meditation is developing inner stillness or *jing*. Inner stillness may be developed through standing, moving, sitting, lying down, and sexual practices. Tai chi as one method of Taoist meditation has the tradition of developing moving stillness (*dong jing*).

In order to achieve maturity and then inner stillness, you will engage in twelve stages of practices to:

1. develop a general ability to focus the mind, until you can keep it concentrated on subtle things beyond mundane tasks. If you can't keep the mind focused steadily on genuine spiritual matters, interest in them too easily becomes a series of fleeting, feel-good, unpleasant, or entertainment experiences
2. explore the meaning of morality (see next section)
3. develop the ability to focus your inner awareness for exceptionally long periods on subtle energetic, mental, or psychic phenomena that may seem invisible or extremely opaque
4. become externally focused on one activity, yet remain internally calm
5. have smooth, unblocked energy channels
6. release, let go, and resolve your inner demons, traumas, and human limitations
7. be calm inside, and yet capable of handling multiple, very intense events without becoming ruffled, or as the Chinese say, you can remain calm and fully present while "riding the whirlwinds"
8. activate the spiritual potential for higher levels of awareness within your internal organs and glands
9. access the ability to use the esoteric five elements that underlie the manifestation of matter and events
10. transcend emotional and psychic negativity that limits your capacity to be balanced and compassionate
11. become capable of truly being in the present moment, and eventually living your life from a timeless place that is beyond past, present, and future
12. develop a mind and spirit that rests in inner stillness, can penetrate to the essence of matters, and see beyond appearances to their roots.

Exploring Spiritual Morality

When tai chi is practiced to achieve inner stillness, one must fully explore the meaning of spiritual morality, known in Chinese as *tao de*—the morals or virtues of the Tao. This begins a strong self-exploration process to find out how morality creates your inner psychic and emotional environment and to recognize its external and internal causes and effects.

Questions naturally arise that demand soul-searching answers. What is virtue? Why be moral? How should morality be expressed? What place should human emotions have in the grand scheme? Should emotions or thoughts be moderated or thrown about with a damn-the-consequences attitude? What is the essential nature of morality, love, compassion, generosity, etc.? If morality is suspended, how does it shred the fabric of your soul and society in general?

Going through this process gives a person a sound footing in their inner world. It cuts the legs off much potential hypocrisy and forestalls needless rebellions that would otherwise drain energy and create problems for delving deeper into spiritual discovery. If morality is omitted from the process, the danger exists that someone may focus purely on gaining power. This often results in making insecurities and spiritual defects even larger, and decreases the potential for transcending them.

Inner Alchemy

The third stage of Taoist meditation, inner alchemy, will not be explored in this book. It is discussed in some detail in Chapter Eight of the second volume of my series on the water method of Taoist meditation: *The Great Stillness*.

Taoist Tai Chi's Meditation Techniques

Taoist meditators believe that as humans each of us have been given three spiritual treasures—our body, the energy which runs our body, and our spirit, called in Chinese *jing, chi,* and *shen* respectively. Each of these spiritual treasures is composed of energy—with body-energy being the least refined and vibrating at the lowest frequency, and spirit-energy being the most refined, vibrating at a much higher frequency.

The overarching initial goal of practicing tai chi as Taoist meditation is to seek and find your spirit, i.e., your soul: that which is permanent and unchanging within you. You then allow your spirit to become fully open and clear, and then bring it to a state of stillness.

In most cases, initially, this is not possible. As a human, your energies at all levels of jing, chi, and shen are blocked from flowing freely and openly. For example, poor physical alignments, blood circulation, or nerve flow can block the optimum functions of the human body.

Closed down acupuncture points, or the inability to store chi-energy in the lower tantien, can block optimum chi-energy flow. Spiritual obstacles can include being excessively self-absorbed, incapable of love, or fearfully consumed by feelings of alienation, morbidity, or events beyond your control.

High-level secular tai chi can be used to unblock the first two treasures of body- and chi-energy. Tai chi, practiced as Taoist moving meditation, is necessary to fully unblock the third treasure of spirit. Taoist tai chi has many specific spiritual meditation techniques to help you do this. Although these will not be covered in detail because they are beyond the scope of this book, a summary follows.

All Taoist meditation methods are based on three major concepts. The first is progressive development from the external, to the more and more internal. The second is resolving body, chi-energy, and spiritual blockages by dissolving or transforming energy. The third is that as you work with the first two ideas, you progressively dig deeper into the core of your being by exploring the interrelationships among the three treasures.

From the External to the Internal: Progressing from Jing (Body) to Chi (Energy) to Shen (Spirit)

In Taoist tai chi, getting the body to function well is the most external aspect; working with subtle chi-energy is more internal; and freeing the spirit is the most internal. Progressively, each is worked on in this order and each sets the foundation for the next. If the foundation set at one stage is weak, then work at the next can be feeble and take longer to accomplish with satisfaction. This is why practitioners must be careful to not attempt to advance too quickly.

Moving From the External: Focus on Jing (Body)

You train your awareness and ability to focus mostly on body techniques, with minimal chi-energy and spirit work, until all your tai chi movements are so natural that you can do them automatically, even if half asleep. You must learn to be able to look straight ahead, and extend your awareness until you can simultaneously feel your entire body *and* see and comprehend what is going on outside it, without lapsing into distracting internal dialogue or "spacing out."

Going Internal: Focus on Chi (Energy)

Your vessel (body) having been prepared, your focus now shifts to how to become aware of, open up, and control all the chi-energies both within your body, and outside it in your external aura. You learn to notice ever more subtle energetic signals, which in turn can lead you to your tensions at the level of spirit. The more strongly your chi-energies flow, the easier it becomes to recognize the experiences lying at the roots of spiritual blockages.

To the Most Internal: Focus on Shen (Spirit)

Here you learn to feel your most internal and refined energies of spirit and resolve the blockages that bind your soul.

Resolving Blockages by Transforming or Dissolving Energy: The Fire and Water Schools of Taoist Meditation

Taoism has fire and water schools of meditation. Both resolve energetic blockages at all levels using energetic techniques from the 16-part nei gung practices (see p. 226), although often with different specifics, rationales, and ways of using intent. The *water schools* emphasize the natural yin path of *allowing, not demanding*, your inner world to change. The *fire schools* emphasize *making things happen* in your inner spiritual world by transforming and controlling energies through conscious focus and will.

In fire methods, resolving blockages is accomplished by deliberately energetically transforming one quality or attitude into another. An example at the spiritual level would be transforming hatred into love, or malaise and paralysis into the capacity for active engagement. The initial central focus within the fire schools is on what is called the micro- and macro-cosmic orbits of energy.

The water schools dissolve or release blockages. The energy becomes empty and neutral of all content. For example, a blockage at your spiritual energy level may cause you to be consistently predisposed toward a negative behavior or feeling. This blockage negates the possibility to freely choose how to behave or feel. If you can dissolve the spiritual energy block, your predispositions will disappear and you can now freely choose and implement how to feel and act.

Whether you use traditional fire or water techniques, as you clear blockages you eventually become conscious of all the physical bodily tissues and all the chi- and spirit-energies that underlie your body. In Taoism this is called "making the body conscious."

The Cyclic Nature of the Three Treasures (Jing, Chi, and Shen)

Once you have a sense of the continuum between the external and internal, you learn to work simultaneously with all three treasures.

You learn to understand how blockages at one energy level can compromise flows at other levels. For example, blockages in your chi-energy channels can deny you full access to the energy of your emotions that run within the same channels. This makes it harder to release and resolve negative emotions such as anger, hate, and paralysis, and replace them with emotions such as patience, compassion, and the willingness to engage. As another example, a block at the level of your spirit, such as malaise, may inhibit the flow of chi-energy in your liver, potentially leading to weakness in the tendons and ligaments of your knees.

These interrelationships create opportunities for spiritual awakening. You can learn to gain access to a blockage at the spiritual level by first learning to recognize and then to resolve a related physical block. Or you can work at the spiritual level to unbind your blocked chi-energy, or vice versa. The three treasures are cyclical. So accessing the body gives access to your chi-energy, which gives maximum access to your spirit, which then gives more access to your body, *ad infinitum*.

During different stages of development, each primary body, chi-energy, or spirit practice either increases or decreases the potential of the other two. For example, say the goal of your moving meditation practice is to work primarily on an aspect of shen (spirit), the last of the three spiritual treasures. If you are attempting to resolve a specific spiritual blockage, you might focus on a specific single *body* mechanism, for example adding specific breath techniques to specific movements, or making micro-movements within your spine, joints, or various internal organs. These or other body parts now become access routes that lead to where the nonphysical spiritual blockage lives in your body. Activating these routes gains you direct access to the spiritual blockage.

The next step is how to awaken the *energy* within these body systems using the energy techniques of the 16-part nei gung system. These amplify energy signatures and allow you to become consciously aware of where they are located and how they can lead you directly and appropriately to the source of your spiritual tensions or blockages. Then spiritual dissolving or transforming techniques can be efficiently applied to resolve the spiritual blockages' underlying source.

As mentioned before, the three treasures are cyclical. Accessing your body gives you access to your chi-energy, which gives maximum access to your spirit, which then gives more access to your body, and so on. With experience, as you clear blockages from each of the three treasures individually, you begin to naturally recognize how to approach and resolve all three simultaneously. This sets off a positive upward spiritual spiral, through which you slowly but surely release and open your spirit and bring it to stillness.

Finding Spirit

As you practice Taoist tai chi, gradually your awareness opens and stabilizes so that you become comfortable staying in the resolved open free space inside you where pure spirit resides. External pressures, and your own internal ones, no longer repeatedly cause you to return to the same blocked places inside you; such pressures no longer trigger old destructive patterns of behavior. Metaphorically, you do not need to scratch familiar old spiritual itches. You achieve longer and longer stable periods of functioning in the new open spiritual space. In a relaxed way spirit begins to feel natural, and you no longer become caught up in the drama of having a "powerful experience" when you meditate. You are beginning to experience spiritual relaxation.

Spiritual Relaxation

Spiritual relaxation is a term Taoists have always used to describe the state of resting in emptiness, in Western parlance where the center of your soul resides. Becoming progressively more spiritually relaxed gives you the opportunity to be open to spirit and thereby enter into profound levels of your being. All the various methods to progressively open the body, chi-energy, and spirit empower each new level of spiritual relaxation. Increased spiritual relaxation allows you to recognize and live from your spiritual essence more and more. Your body, energy, and thoughts flow directly into the source of your spirit within and settle there.

Connecting to Your Essence and the Tao

When your spiritual tensions release and fully relax, your inner world unites. Your inner sense of being composed of multiple parts, which many experience, ceases. A stable, non-expressible essence emerges, which now becomes the cornerstone of your spiritual life. This is when

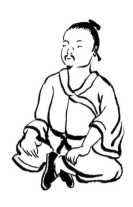

answers spontaneously emerge to fundamental spiritual questions, such as "Who am I?" and "What is my place in the universe?" Your unique individual essence now becomes obvious, and transcends all qualities of personality or personal history.

To the Taoist way of spiritual thinking it is only from this level of awareness that it becomes possible to truly begin to understand and walk the Path of the Tao—the road that connects all and everything.

Taoist Tai Chi and Spiritual Stress

The ordinary stress that people experience from excessive work and family pressures is endemic in Western culture. Spiritual stress has deeper and more existential roots.

Fundamental spiritual questions naturally arise in people, be they religious or not. Much to the amazement of parents, even young children, without any prompting, will ask existential questions: What happens when I die? Why am I alive? What am I here for? What's life all about? Ultimately, logic alone can't give true satisfaction, as these questions truly have no definitive, black-and-white answers.

At all stages of life, unsatisfying answers to these questions can lead people into dark nights of the soul and shaky self-doubt. As there are no true answers, this can create immense internal stress, the causes of which are not easily identified. When people are in the midst of a spiritual crisis, it may take them some time to recognize and resolve what is wrong. The capacity to find some source within, some ever-flowing wellspring of spiritual strength and equanimity, is the only buffer against deep spiritual stress.

Secular tai chi can help you deal with ordinary stress. Only Taoist tai chi or some other deep meditation or religious practice can help you with spiritual stress.

The Causes of Spiritual Stress

Unresolved blocked spiritual tensions create spiritual stress. Resolving them requires you first to become aware of these tensions, and then fully relax them. Spiritual tension causes the innermost recesses of your soul to contract and become frozen. If these tensions become severe enough they result in spiritual alienation and malaise. This makes life a burden to be carried rather than a wonderful journey to be engaged in with joy and reverence.

If your innermost being contracts and shuts down, you may feel as though you are slowly dying. But only you can know to what degree spiritual tension resides inside you and the extent to which it is affecting you.

Here are some questions to ask in order to take stock of your life:

- Do love and compassion seem to be deserting your life of their own accord, not just because you are temporarily feeling angry or rejected?
- Has life boiled down to only grasping after your self-interests?
- Are you becoming numb inside?
- Are you ceasing to connect to anything alive in a meaningful way?
- Are inner dread and paralysis becoming normal?
- Are you blinded to the wonders of creation, great or small?

It is the author's observation that on a macro level spiritual malaise lies at the heart of many ills that plague society. We have many of the practical abilities and resources to cure many of those ills, such as healing the environment or reducing poverty. So far we have not made a commitment to do so, not because we lack love, compassion, or kindness, but because we lack the will and follow-through that spiritual malaise so often saps. Life and stress seem to exponentially speed up. Just taking care of family and business life soaks up most people's time and energies. Most just scramble to keep up, leaving no time for spiritual reflection.

Secular tai chi will relieve and slow down the stresses of ordinary life and prepare you to explore a spiritual path. However, only true meditation has the potential to cure the deeper roots of spiritual malaise, so endemic in Western culture.

Spiritual Stress and the Elderly
Many elderly people feel spiritual stress. After living a full life with many experiences, there are often many real and imagined reasons for regrets, especially as the end draws undeniably near. Endlessly churning over these regrets can exacerbate all your negative stress mechanisms, potentially causing disease, reducing your life span, and stealing life's joy.

Taoist tai chi and other form of meditation help reduce spiritual stress. Finding a spiritual center allows your body to let go of the past, and your mind to slow down and cease churning. It encourages your internal focus to shift toward cherishing and remembering all that is wonderful in your life. It predisposes you to look forward to ways to make life better, rather than remembering how spiritually unsatisfying it has been. Successful resolution to spiritual stress is an essential part of any longevity program. Taoism and Taoist tai chi pay close attention to it.

Spiritual Tension Can Result in Poor Health

Spiritual tension can make your spirit ill in its deepest recesses.

Some confuse deeper spiritual tensions with ordinary poor physical or psychological health. Conversely, others may falsely think that the ultimate cause of a mundane illness is spiritual or karmic, therefore allowing them to blame themselves or others for being ill.

Both spiritual and mundane illness can arise simultaneously and be inseparably intertwined. Improving or worsening either one can exacerbate or mitigate the experiences and symptoms of the other. The body or emotions can still remain ill after spiritual issues are dealt with. Or the body-mind can be well while the spirit is ill—or both can feed on each other in a corrosive dance where both partners hold each other tight and squeeze the life out of each other.

Taoist Tai Chi Requires Regular Practice

Taoist tai chi can help reduce spiritual stress, but only if you practice regularly. After establishing a period of regular daily practice, throughout a normal day when not doing tai chi you will become able to recognize the emergence of spiritual blockages in very visceral energetic ways. Time permitting, you can practice tai chi to resolve these blocks, preventing them from accumulating and activating a downward stress cycle. Tai chi becomes a regular spiritual metronome. It creates deep internal rhythms to keep you constantly aware of spirit.

In the beginning, the ability to incorporate spiritual practices attained during tai chi into other aspects of your life will be relatively difficult. Over time, however, this changes. Gradually in times other than practicing tai chi, you start strongly recognizing within your thoughts a sense of subtle chi-energy when a blockage is actively emerging that needs to be dispersed before it unravels your life that day. Ultimately, even without outward movements, during all times and circumstances you can use Taoist tai chi's inner techniques to immediately resolve spiritual blockages when you recognize them emerging. Reducing both spiritual and ordinary stress often defuses potentially destructive situations.

Conclusion

Secular tai chi can help your mind and body relax and achieve the quietness that many people associate with spirituality. These qualities help build the foundation for all forms of traditional meditation.

In Taoist meditation, the goal of spirituality is to connect with the deepest recesses of your being and consciousness (the Tao). This spiritual path requires commitment to both learning and practicing.

Within tai chi, there is a rare tradition that teaches you to use tai chi to achieve the goals of Taoist meditation (Taoist tai chi). These goals are achieved in three stages: maturity, inner stillness, and inner alchemy.

9 Choosing a Tai Chi Style

Essentially all tai chi styles have far more in common with each other than they have differences. All improve health, reduce stress, and help you move more gracefully. All develop chi, and use slow-motion, flowing, circular movements. As an art of living, tai chi engenders a powerful creative process that from moment to moment allows us to express our innermost selves.

In the perception of most beginners, the importance of styles does not register. Few say, "I want to learn such and such a tai chi style," and then go find someone who teaches it. Few understand what the differences are and how they might matter. For most, the style taught is less important than the quality of the teacher, the convenience of the school, and so on.

Moreover, many tai chi students become emotionally invested in the first style they learned, without understanding how it fits within the entire context of tai chi. If they had known, they might have chosen a style more appropriate to their goals rather than just walking into the first tai chi class they came across.

Besides finding a good teacher, three issues should be paramount in your decision-making process when choosing a tai chi style (these issues will be treated in some detail in this chapter so that you will have enough basic information to help you better make the most appropriate choices):

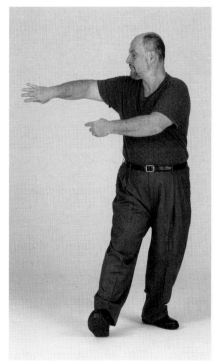

Guy Hearn

Wu style tai chi transition movement within Fair Lady Weaves the Shuttles. This move is unique to the Wu style long form

- Which style? There are five main ones—Yang, Wu, Chen, Hao, and combination styles
- Which frame? Each style has various size frames—small, medium, and large. This choice can be even more important than the style
- Which form? Forms within each style are of different lengths—short, medium, and long—and these forms may be similar or radically different.

Each style has a different syllabus, structure, and flavor as regards how its specific techniques are applied. All five styles can potentially give you tai chi's health benefits. However, in the beginning years of learning, knowing something about the different approaches is important because of the different effects they can have on your body, mind, and spirit.

Tai Chi's Five Major Styles

Tai chi has five major styles—Yang, Wu, Chen, Hao, and combination styles. Except for the combination styles, each derives its name from the founder's surname. The Chinese talk about the tai chi of the Yang Family, Wu Family, Chen Family, and Hao Family.

Each style takes a different approach toward the movements of their forms, and each style has many variations or schools. Each school is composed of practitioners who follow specific leaders or teachers within the style. Each school emphasizes a specific approach to the art: their forms may have recognizable stylistic differences, trademark movements, or develop specific self-defense training skills. Although embodying the same principles, a posture with the same name may look different in different styles. This can be seen in the following pictures.

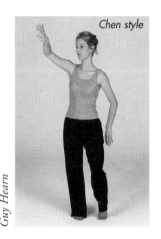
Chen style

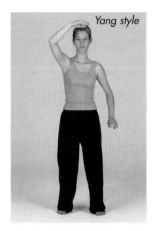
Yang style

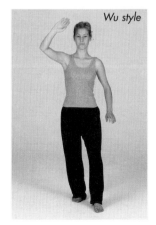
Wu style

Guy Hearn

White Crane Spreads its Wings

Although the variations make for wonderful points of debate and gossip, if your primary goal is health and longevity, these differences probably won't matter much. However, if you do tai chi for self-defense or high performance, it is important that your teacher, whatever style he or she teaches, includes some degree of internal chi-work in order for you to get the maximum benefit from your tai chi practice.

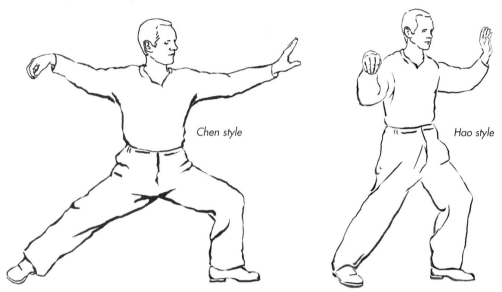

Chen style

Hao style

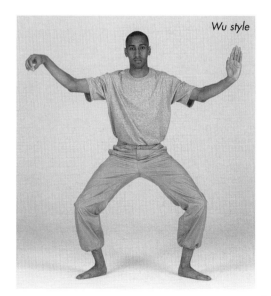

Wu style

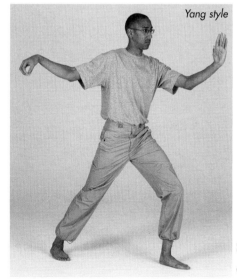

Yang style

Single Whip

Guy Hearn

Although some kind of tai chi is taught in most small towns in the West, only in the largest cities with large Chinese populations will you find all styles being offered. The relative geographical prevalence of each of the styles in the West has been mostly a function of which Chinese immigrants showed up first in which locations, where they came from in China, and if they openly taught tai chi or not. Cultural advances in general tend to spread out more from big cities than from sparsely populated areas.

The Yang Style

The Yang style is the most popular and widely practiced tai chi style worldwide. In England and America, at least 20 main variations of Yang style exist, and in China even more. The various schools originated from the approach of a specific master or from a particular geographic region within China. Each variation has a distinct flavor, looks different from the others to a greater or lesser degree, and may emphasize some different technical points. All, however, will be called Yang style.

The Wu Style

The Wu style is the second most popular style. It has three main variations, with strong stylistic differences that derived from the founder, Chuan You, his son, Wu Jien Chuan, and his grandchildren. The Wu style was created directly from the Yang and as such is the largest variant of the Yang style. However, unlike most traditions in the Yang style, most Wu schools emphasize small, compact movements over large and medium-sized ones.[1]

The Yang and Wu, with all their variations, encompass the vast majority (80 percent or more) of all tai chi practitioners.

The Chen Village Style

The Chen village style is the original style of tai chi from which the Yang style was created. It is relatively hard to find Chen style teachers, and adherents account for about one percent of tai chi practitioners.

Unlike most tai chi, not all the movements of its first level of training are initially done in slow motion. The Chen style alternates slow-motion movements with short, fast, explosive ones. It demands more physical coordination and may strain the lower back and knees more than other styles; consequently it is difficult for the elderly or injured to learn. The complexity of its movements, which include fast releases combined with jumping kicks and stamping actions, makes

---

[1] However, in contrast to the Yang style norm, Master William C. C. Chen does a Yang style that also has very high stances and relatively small style movements.

it more athletic and physically difficult than most other tai chi styles, and as such, often more appealing to young people.

Today, many of the Chen style's better teachers learned in the Chen village itself or from the village's most accomplished member, Chen Fa Ke, who taught in Beijing in the first half of the twentieth century. Within the Chen village itself, and nearby, there was both a large frame tai chi style (with large extended movements that the founder of the Yang style learned) and a small frame style (called the Zhao Bao), which the founder of the Hao style learned.

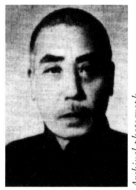

Archival photograph

Chen Fa Ke (1887–1957), father of the modern Chen style and the first major Chen teacher to come out of the Chen village and teach in Beijing

The Hao Style

The Hao style is exceedingly rare in China and almost non-existent in the West. Its small frame movements are extremely small. Its primary focus is on tai chi's more internal chi movements, with physical motions being much less important. As such it is considered an advanced style that is hard to appreciate for practitioners without significant background knowledge of tai chi.

Combination Styles

Combination styles are the third most popular styles after the Yang and the Wu. These styles freely mix and match movements from the four other tai chi styles, as well as movements from other internal martial arts styles such as ba gua and hsing-i. Sometimes they may even add movements from Shaolin kung fu, Chinese wrestling, or other martial arts. Combination styles are primarily done in slow motion.

The combination styles you are most likely to find in the West include the Sun style, which combined Hao tai chi with ba gua and hsing-i; the Fu style, which combined Yang tai chi with ba gua and hsing-i; the Kuang Ping Yang style developed by Guo Lien Ying, which has a strong hsing-i and ba gua flavor; and the Chen Pan Ling style, which combines Yang, Wu, and Chen tai chi with ba gua, hsing-i, and Shaolin kung fu.

Secret Styles

In addition to the above styles, there are those that are said to be "secret styles." Teachers claim they existed before the Chen village style or were derived from someone who had learned it in secret from one of the founders or close associates of the founders of the four main styles.

Regardless of whether or not a given secret style is of inferior or superior quality, most were fairly recently created, despite the usual claim of having originated in the untraceable distant past. This is because within Chinese society, being ancient conferred authenticity and valuable marketing advantages. The quality of these styles normally depends on whether the person who made the claims had a high level of skill or not. Generally, however, most of these "secret styles" are in reality combination styles.

History of the Tai Chi Styles

Many tai chi books go into great detail about the numerous specifics relating to the creation of the different tai chi styles and their most prominent masters. Here is a summary.

What we currently know as tai chi was first established in the seventeenth century in central China's Chen village, according to the verifiable facts available today. Before then, the Taoist internal energy principles, upon which tai chi is based, existed in oral traditions and in published form since the tenth century.

The most common pre-Chen village mythology states that the Taoist sage Chang San Feng created some form of tai chi after being inspired by watching a battle between a snake and a crane. He created a soft internal martial art that infused within it the wisdom, military strategies, and longevity methods of Taoism.

How tai chi was established in the Chen family village is still being debated along two lines of thought. According to the first theory, a Chen village headman (Chen Wan Ting) created tai chi by collating various martial arts techniques he learned outside the village when he was an army general. According to the second, a mysterious stranger named Wang Tsung Yueh, arrived at the Chen village, where he taught a version of tai chi that he learned from one of several possible lineages that may have derived from Chang San Feng. Wang infused the Taoist internal energy work into the village's existing martial art (which is clearly recognizable as what the village headman learned in the army) and fused them together.

The Chen village kept tai chi a closely guarded secret for over a century and refused to teach it to a single outsider. Having a superior martial art enabled the village to stay safe from marauding bandits and safely conduct business without their goods being stolen or having to pay protection money. The villagers, however, developed this internal martial art to a very high level.

In the nineteenth century, an immensely talented and moti-vated young man with a great love of martial arts, by the name of Yang Lu Chan, was told by his teacher that if he wanted to progress, he needed to go to the Chen village. At this point the story becomes an inspiring one about true grit, perseverance, and humility in the pursuit of excellence.

Yang went to Chen village, asked to be admitted and was summarily refused. The teachings were secret and forbidden to non-family members. Yang devised an immensely disciplined strategy. Posing as a deaf-mute, he obtained work as a servant in the house of the teaching master. A diligent and cheerful worker, over time he became trusted enough to be given free reign of the house, including the keys to the locked doors surrounding the training hall. Keeping himself hidden, he secretly watched the classes and practiced late into the night when everyone was asleep, no doubt overcoming years of sleep deprivation to succeed.

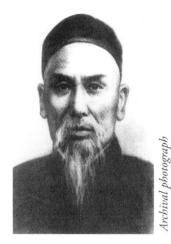

Yang Lu Chan (1799–1872) who brought the secrets of tai chi out of the Chen village into the modern world and founded the Yang style

Archival photograph

At the time, the Chen teaching master had a dilemma. The next generation of the village was resting on the family laurels and not training sufficiently. The master was greatly concerned and saddened, and feared that his family's art of tai chi would be lost.

One night Yang was caught. He was dragged down to the training hall. The students, not wishing their position to be usurped, demanded his execution for breaching security—a rea-sonable response in nineteenth-century China given the circumstances.

Speaking for the first time, Yang profusely apologized. A shocked Chen master then pon-dered the implications of the discipline required to maintain this deaf-mute act for years. Yang begged the Chen master to be allowed to learn his art. He then challenged his would-be executioners and, one by one, using their own techniques, Yang managed to defeat them.

The master, who was truly searching for a good student to pour his knowledge into, won-dered what Yang could do if he got the full meal rather than only the crumbs. After a psycho-logically grueling three-day test of character, Chen accepted Yang for what ultimately became an 18-year apprenticeship. After completing the full training, Yang left the village with his teacher's blessing to go out into the world and teach however he thought fit.

After this Yang traveled around and challenged China's best martial arts exponents. He convincingly defeated all of them without injuring anyone, a sign of truly remarkable skill. Gradually he found his way to the imperial capital Beijing, did the same there, and became the teacher of the imperial guards and many aristocrats.

Although most wealthy aristocrats were not fighters, they found that the tai chi's energy work did wonders for their health and general vitality. In order to make it more accessible to them, and others, Yang simplified the complex movements of the Chen style, and thereby created the Yang style. The methods taught by Yang and his son (Yang Pan Hou) are called the Old Yang style, and are relatively rare. The style taught by his grandson (Yang Cheng Fu) is called the New Yang style, which is practiced by the vast majority of Yang style practitioners today.

Yang Lu Chan had a student named Wu Yu Hsiang, who was a governmental official. After studying with Yang, he decided to learn directly from Yang's master in the Chen village. On the way there, however, he was diverted to a nearby village and spent a long time learning the small frame Chen style from a different Chen master. During this same period Wu also discovered a thin volume called the *Tai Chi Classics*, languishing in a corner of a salt store. This volume contains all the principles, albeit in very terse form, upon which tai chi is based (see p. 237).

By combining Yang's teachings and the small frame Chen style, Wu created the Hao style. It was initially called the Wu Yu Hsiang style, but because Wu did not have a male descendant, it was renamed after one of his relatives, Hao Wei Zhen. Today it is called the Hao style—the name this book will use so as not to confuse it with the different and more popular Wu style, which is described next, and the Yang and Chen styles, from which it was entirely derived. The Hao style is the smallest frame tai chi style.

The Chen style is the first generation tai chi style, while the Yang and Hao are second generation. The third generation of tai chi is the Wu style. The Wu style was developed by Yang's best student in the imperial guards, Chuan You, who was highly skilled in the small frame aspect of Yang's teaching. The Wu style was further refined and completed by Chuan You's son, Wu Jien Chuan, who learned both from his father and from Yang's son, Pan Hou, also a small frame adept. Wu Jien Chuan taught in the Yang family association in Beijing and later

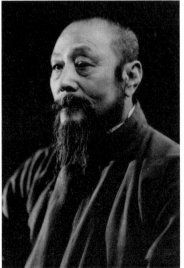

Wu Jien Chuan (1870–1942), co-founder of the Wu style of tai chi

spread his method all over China. Being 20 years older, Wu had quite an influence on Yang's grandson Yang Cheng Fu, who created what is called the New Yang style. Through their collaboration their forms have the same basic structure.

Mixing and matching techniques from the earlier tai chi styles created the fourth generation of tai chi styles—the combination styles—during the first half of the twentieth century.

Large, Medium, and Small Frame Styles

Each style has versions with different frame sizes. (The term frame is used in the sense of the size of a picture frame. Smaller physical movements fit in smaller frames; larger ones need larger frames.) A frame may be looked at from two basic perspectives.

1. **How large you make your external movements.**

   In large frame styles, you will do large, clean, obvious extended arm movements, with large waist turns and long deep stances. Small frame styles condense the movements, using relatively small and subtly intricate arm movements, medium to small waist turns and shorter stances. These shorter stances usually stand higher, although they can go as low as the most stretched-out large frame stances.

   In a large frame style movement, your hand, wrist, or elbow may move thirty inches in space; but only five to ten inches in a similar small frame style. In large and medium frame styles, your waist may turn a full 90 degrees completely to the side; but only half that amount, to 45 degrees, or less in a small frame style

2. **How you develop chi.**

   Large frame styles emphasize correct external movements and naturally focus your attention to the space outside yourself. The initial strategy is to focus your attention on the muscles, tendons, and alignments needed to maintain your skeleton's structural integrity. It does so in order to ultimately influence your deeper bodily systems and the creation of chi within you. In tai chi, this is called "the outside opens the inside," or "from the external to the internal."

   Small frame styles use a more internal approach. They emphasize correct movement of chi through the deeper internal systems inside your body (spine, internal organs, spaces within the joints, etc.) to create correct and efficient physical movements and body alignments. The nature of the smaller external movements tends to focus your attention inwardly, for example into your internal organs. In tai chi this is called "the inside opens the outside," or "from the internal to the external."

Some people and body types may prefer the long extended movements of large frame styles; others may find tighter, less extended, close movements of medium and smaller frame styles more appropriate. It is slightly more common for long-limbed body types to gravitate toward the extended movements of large frame styles, and for those with shorter limbs or a longer torso to prefer small and medium frame styles. Both beginners and relatively experienced practitioners may subliminally react to what they are being taught with a sense of comfort or indefinable unease, depending on whether their bodies are doing large, medium, or small frame tai chi.

The Continuum Between Small, Medium, and Large Frame Styles Shown Using the Tai Chi Movement Push Downward

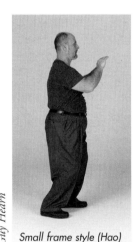 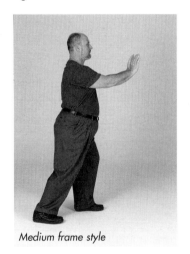 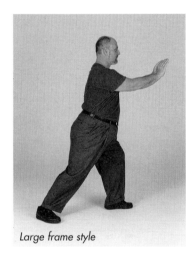

Small frame style (Hao)   Medium frame style   Large frame style

Guy Hearn

Although all frame styles stretch the muscles and make the body more flexible, the large frame strategy is to focus on outer stretching, that is, getting your hands and feet to extend farther and farther away from your torso. Just as in a leg split, the lower you go the more you stretch. However, deeper, longer stances may aggravate the knees and back.

Small frame styles focus more on inner stretching, i.e., releasing internal organs and ligaments, while increasing the spaces between your vertebrae and within your joints, without extending your hands and feet very far away from your torso. This process stretches the muscles by reducing the internal anatomical pulls and involuntary nervous system contractions that prevent muscles from naturally stretching, so they release and effortlessly elongate. Small frame styles also gradually enable you to become both very relaxed and extremely limber. Moreover, they make it easier to open the body's acupuncture meridians and other deeper internal energy channels.

Small styles have an inner orientation and tend to release bound or stagnant energy faster. They make it easier for you to focus on the inner emotional realities you live with on a daily basis, either consciously or unconsciously. If you are not yet willing to deal with what is negatively impacting your psyche, then small styles could be discomforting. Not everyone wants to feel or understand what's inside them in order to iron out the rough edges and overcome what is spiritually limiting their lives. As the old joke goes, Da Nile (denial) is not just a river in Egypt. However, for those who have the courage to look inside, all you will find is what is actually in there—the good, the bad, the ugly, and the potential of all you can be.

Large frame styles have a more outer orientation. They can give you the health benefits and mitigate the stresses in your life, but do not tend to emphasize any psychologically unpleasant subliminal pressures, which you may have not yet dealt with, and may not wish to.

A specific school within a style may teach only the techniques and principles of one specific frame (large, medium, or small) to the exclusion of all others. Alternatively, a student may be first trained in a large frame manner until their chi grows sufficiently strong. Then the teacher will introduce more sophisticated adjustments in a graduated continuum that will progress from large to medium to small frame ways of doing the same tai chi movements. Eventually, the student may be shown how to combine the small, medium, and large frame techniques into various applications.

Long, Medium, and Short Forms

Which form is best for you? Within each individual style, forms have fewer or greater numbers of movements that may differ slightly or dramatically from each other.

Each style contains a number of individual or repeated movements (postures) called a form or set. All of its moves are strung together with smooth transitions in a seamless continuous flow, without starts, stops, or jerky movements.

Medium and short forms originate from their style's long form. Short forms usually have 15 to 40 movements; medium forms between 40 and 70, and long forms 80 movements or more.

After forms reach a certain number of movements, specific moves repeat, with each repetition counted as a separate movement within the total number, for example 88, 108, or 128.

For health and stress reduction, most forms are done at various slow-motion speeds. Although the overwhelming majority of tai chi schools only teach slow-motion forms, a few from all tai chi styles teach forms that alternate slow-motion moves with fast ones.

The Relative Advantages of Short, Medium, and Long Forms

Generally, the longer a form, the deeper it works its benefits into your body and the greater the commitment it demands. Shorter forms require less commitment from you in terms of practice and learning.

Short Forms

It is my opinion, after having taught thousands of tai chi students worldwide, that most beginners are better served starting off with a short form. It is more likely you will finish a short form than a long form. After a little grounding in the art, it is more likely you may acquire the interest and desire to learn longer forms.

Short forms provide most of the essential broad benefits tai chi can offer, although not to the same degree as the longer forms. You obtain the real experience of doing tai chi without having to make a major commitment. Short forms take less time to learn. The sequences are easier to remember, which is ideal for older people who may be beginning to experience memory problems.

Many find the physical coordination needed to do a tai chi form to be as, or more difficult, than feeling or moving chi. For them, learning a smaller number of movements is an easier road to gaining the benefits of letting go of physical tension, calming the mind, and getting into their chi.

For a stronger workout, simply move more and more slowly, or repeat your form over and over again. To gain maximum benefit, keep moving continuously between repetitions, without stopping or resting in between.

Medium-length Forms

Medium-length forms of between 40 and 70 movements are most commonly found in the Yang and Chen styles. They tend to contain most, although not necessarily all the postures (moves) of a long form. They don't repeat specific postures as many times as long forms do. Because they have significantly more individual movements than short forms, they challenge your physical coordination skills more, but require less stamina and time than long forms.

Medium-length forms are better than short ones in terms of the number of different postures, which reach deeper into the body, and thereby stretch more specific soft tissue—tendons, ligaments, and fasciae—and increase different ranges of motion for specific parts of your body. Energetically, each new and different individual posture also provides added benefits to your whole body's chi circulation.

Long Forms

Long forms provide tai chi's maximum benefits. Long forms are designed to exponentially increase the flow of chi at regular intervals during the form. Unlike short forms, the long forms of the Yang, Wu, and combination styles are broken into three clear sections.[2] At the end of each movement phase, your energy revs up to a higher level. In other words, the more movements there are, the bigger volume of energy you accrue per minute of your practice routine. There is an even bigger jump experienced in energy accrual when you do a long form's second and final sections.

Contained within the techniques of long forms is the complete tai chi martial art technology, including overall strategies and types of internal power development. The techniques can be easily adapted by athletes, who wish to learn tai chi to increase performance in their chosen sport.

Long forms require the most work, commitment, and perseverance and are initially more difficult to learn. Some find it hard to remember what move comes next, especially if they do not have someone to follow in front of them or they have not practiced for a while. Long forms usually include some postures absent in medium forms, and normally are a more intense workout than either short or medium forms. The combination of these factors can make long forms too hard for the less patient beginner.

Long and medium forms can also function as short forms if only the first section of movements are performed; these take up approximately the same time as a very short form.

How Long Does it Take to Do a Form?

For health and stress reduction, the forms are done at four degrees of slow-motion speed. From start to finish, using a standard baseline of a 108-movement long form, a moderately fast degree of slow motion would need 15 minutes; slow motion, 25 minutes; very slow 45 minutes; and a super-slow speed an hour or more. A short form can range from between three and twenty minutes to complete, depending on the number of movements and your practice speed.

---

[2] A notable exception is the Yang short form of the Cheng Man Ching school, which also includes three clear sections.

Push Hands

All styles of tai chi include push hands. It is a bridge between the tai chi form and tai chi's self-defense skills. In this generally non-violent semi-sparring exercise, two people's arms remain in constant contact, as they try to unbalance and push each other without resorting to overt muscular force.

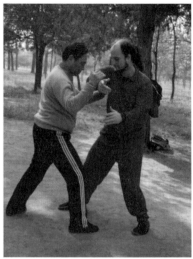

In tai chi, it is often said that the solo form is for understanding yourself, and push hands is for understanding others. Push hands challenges and tests your inner perceptions. Like a mirror, it shows whether you can translate the form's basic principles and movements into real life human interactions, either for human relationships, physical self-defense or stress management. Some tai chi teachers will bring some form of gentle, non-threatening push hands into their classes because it is an effective tool for training relaxation. Moreover, in its more common gentle incarnations, push hands is a

Chen style master, Feng Zhi Qiang, and the author doing Fixed Push Hands. *Feng was the youngest disciple of Chen Fa Ke, from whom the modern Chen style of tai chi originated*

tremendous tool for removing the habits ingrained in your nervous system that trigger stress. It can provide valuable training to help prevent injuries caused by intense physical strain.

However, only about half of tai chi teachers in the West regularly teach some type of push hands and the quality of instruction varies. Relatively few teach push hands as a serious part of a realistic self-defense program, but many teach it for health and stress reduction.

For more information on push hands, see Chapter 7.

The Best Style for Improving Health and Managing Stress

For healing, the styles that are done in slow motion tend to be more effective. The Chen style's emphasis on explosive movements regularly interspersed throughout the form can jar the joints and spine. This tends to make it less effective for healing in general, and for back problems specifically.

All styles work equally well for healing musculoskeletal and internal organs problems due to weakness or energetic imbalance.

For problems caused by external physical, chemical, or psychological trauma, the small frame, more internal styles tend to be more effective. This is due to their ability to release stored energy deep in the body which normal movement alone usually will not unravel and release.

The Best Style for Beginners

If a style is naturally more comfortable and easier for you to learn and remember, you are more likely to finish learning it, remember the order of the moves, and practice it on your own. That said, the following points should be considered when choosing a style:

- The physical coordination skills of the Yang, Wu, and Hao styles are usually the easiest to learn, the combination styles are in the middle, and the Chen style is the most difficult
- If your body is extremely tight and your goal is to get stretched out, the large styles of tai chi will initially work faster, especially for the legs and hips. However, the smaller styles will also get the same job done over time
- For those with a bad lower back or injured knees, forms with higher, rather than lower stances are better. Smaller frame styles tend to have higher stances
- Large styles initially make it easier to develop leg strength, because of their longer and deeper stances
- Smaller styles make it easier to access the more internal work tai chi has to offer, including making it easier to work directly with the internal organs.

Why Learn Tai Chi Instead of Another Discipline?

Whether anyone should do one discipline or another is a matter of personal choice. Different approaches may be appropriate at different points of life. Tai chi doesn't say, "If you do tai chi, you can't or shouldn't do that." It tends to look at the potential consequences if you do the something else. For example, exercises based on physical tension can make your body feel dead or numb, neither of which will make you feel more relaxed and alive. Alternatively, the more capable you are of relaxing, the more you can tense either your body or mind if that is what you need or desire for other activities. Conversely, tension does not enhance your ability to relax; rather it inhibits it, especially after the tension becomes habitual.

Tai chi can make your body and mind more relaxed, and your energy more smooth, balanced, and strong. The more you can relax your mind, the more you can focus with stamina and without easily becoming distracted. Tai chi complements most other body practices:

- Both *aerobics* and tai chi improve circulation, albeit in different ways (see Chapter 5). Tai chi movements are more varied than non-impact aerobics and are more likely to fully engage the mind and thus avoid eventual boredom.
- All *martial arts*, in different ways, to varying capacities and over different periods of time, teach useable self-defense skills. Some will make you fitter than tai chi. Few, however, will also maintain your health or help to heal your injuries or medical problems as well as tai chi.

  Some people find that external martial arts, such as karate and kung fu, can create aggression. Doing tai chi can mitigate this. Other external martial artists often simply want to add effective soft and circular martial techniques not fully present in their own styles. Some find the philosophy of softness overcoming hardness, with all its hidden and subtle aspects, more in line with the way their personality would like to do martial arts or competitive sports. The difference between how linear and circular martial arts techniques work either for combat, sports, or for emotional and spiritual health is profound.
- In many ways tai chi and serious *weight training* are complete opposites. When two things are opposites their appeals lie in different areas. Any debate about better or worse ultimately comes down to whether you prefer yin or yang, internal or external fitness, a

debate beyond the scope of this book—tai chi is firmly in the yin corner, weightlifting in the yang.

As a complementary practice tai chi can loosen up the excessively tight muscles and improve rotation in the joints that weight lifters may have lost, thereby restoring more fluid body motion. A lack of range of motion may make people muscle bound and more prone to injuries, such as torn muscles.

The Best Style for People Over Fifty

The slow motion, short form styles are generally best for people over age fifty because they take longer to learn movements than younger people. Therefore, beginning with a short form, and learning a long form later on, if desired, is a less frustrating and easier path for older people to enjoy, absorb, and remember tai chi.

The Chen style is not usually recommended for older beginners, because of its stamping, jumping, and sudden moves. The small frame styles (Wu and Hao) generally have higher stances than the large frame styles. For older people with weak or injured lower backs or knees, forms with higher, rather than lower stances are better. Deeper, longer stances, more common in large frame styles, can aggravate the knees and back. But if your knees are already strong, deeper, longer stances can make your legs stronger at a faster speed. The small frame styles are usually better for upgrading the health of your internal organs.

The most important thing is to find a patient instructor who does not judge or put expectations on you in terms of how fast or how precisely you should be learning the moves. For most older people, the bigger movements of large frame styles may be easier to remember initially, and the smaller styles more fascinating once you have some tai chi background.

Conclusion

Tai chi can be a friend for life. Knowing the various perspectives and frameworks in which tai chi is taught will help you choose a style appropriate to your goals, age, and learning abilities.

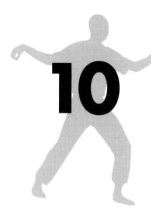

10 Beginning Students:

What You Can Expect to Learn

During my 11 years of study in China, I never met or observed a person who had a higher level of skill in the internal martial arts than Liu Hung Chieh of Beijing, a renowned tai chi and meditation master and lineage holder. One day, after watching the eighty-year-old Liu do his tai chi form, I asked him what it was like to do it perfectly.

He considered the question for a while, gently smiled and replied,

"I don't know, I am still waiting to find out. I have practiced internal martial arts virtually every day of my life for over seventy years, including tai chi for over fifty. One day, maybe twenty years ago, it seemed I did the tai chi form perfectly. It was a very good feeling. Then a few days later it was obvious I hadn't.

"I can say as the years have gone by, that it has been possible to do the form better, more efficiently, and with deeper satisfaction. However, no matter how good it gets, after a while something a little more interesting usually happens. Young man, humans are humans, and gods are gods. Gods maybe can be perfect, humans rarely. Practice regularly. Do your best moment by moment, and tai chi will give back to you more than you can possibly give to it. Relax, do, and let the beauty of the art unfold."

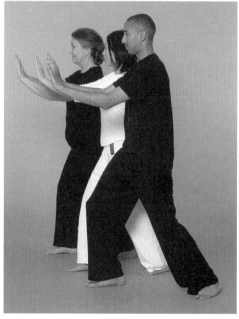

Guy Hearn

The tai chi posture Push Downwards, variations of which repeat many times in all tai chi forms

Time has shown me through personal experience that his words were very true.

Realistic Expectations

After thirty years of teaching tai chi, I have found that many people, after truly benefiting from doing tai chi, quit. They do so because they had false expectations that were impossible to fulfill, and disinformation about what should or should not be happening to themselves or others. Perhaps this chapter will help you recognize the more realistic benefits and challenges of learning tai chi, so that you will be more likely to stick with it longer and benefit more.

False expectations can come from many places. For example, you may feel that learning tai chi will make you a superhero, like those in the exaggerated world of entertainment fiction, with its inspiring stories of the feats of spiritual super-beings that are so far from where humans can start, or even finish in their lifetime.

Or you might have false expectations from reading some of the texts of tai chi literature, where it is easy to misinterpret and blur the lines between fact, inspiration, and metaphor. Many Westerners lack sufficient background knowledge to fully appreciate either the complete or specific context of these literary statements and what their subtext does or does not imply.

Here are some points to ponder when you are thinking about learning tai chi:

- Tai chi is challenging to learn. People who do tai chi well make it look easy and effortless. But the truth is tai chi is not especially easy to learn. An interesting point about learning anything of value, including tai chi, is "things are difficult when you can't and easy after you can"
- The road to attaining such a wonderful degree of fluid, smooth, and relaxed movements requires much patience and effort, just as any sport or art form
- Tai chi requires, and progressively develops, tremendous amounts of both gross and subtle physical coordination. Although quite "doable," this can frustrate those who perceive themselves to be coordinated as much as those who consider themselves uncoordinated. Tai chi is one of the most sophisticated methods of integrated whole-body movement that humans have so far created. All parts of your body are supposed to move together, at the same relative speed. In all movements, no matter how tiny, ideally each

individual joint is directly and simultaneously linked to and moves in coordination with every other joint in the body

- Tai chi is a workout that can be as strenuous and invigorating as aerobics, even though it can look so easy, simple, and relaxed. You are going to use muscles that you didn't know you had. Before you really learn to relax and soften your body, the habitual tension stored in your legs and shoulders may make you tremble and ache. At most points in time, most physical activities focus on only a few muscle groups working to their maximum, with the majority of your muscles doing relatively little. In tai chi, every muscle, no matter how small, is supposed to move and exert the same effort relative to its size as the biggest muscles

- It is quite normal to feel some emotional unpleasantness, especially as you begin to really notice, often for the first time, what stress is doing to your nervous system, or how unquiet and devoid of inner peace your mind and emotions really are. For everyone, part of learning tai chi is learning to recognize the subtle tensions within your body and mind. This can "freak you out" as you may not be able to believe the degree of unconscious tension you and virtually everyone else you know holds. Although practice empowers you to learn to let go of your physical tension, it can be a real shock to recognize each more profound personal level of emotional and mental tension hidden beneath

- At first, it may be difficult to practice on your own. It is best not to feel guilty about this; just accept your limitations rather than quitting

- Your sense of progress will not be a constant upward curve. Tai chi tends to be more of a zigzag, with peaks, valleys, and plateaus. Tai chi is not a get-rich-quick kind of thing, applied to health. Rather it is a get-rich-slowly exercise, which is how finance really works most of the time

- Different people prefer to learn in different ways. Some simply want to follow the leader and mimic the movements. Others wish to be taught why they are doing what they are doing and how to use it in their lives. If you expect one but get the other, you need to change either your expectations or your teacher

- It is initially difficult to understand, much less feel, the benefits of practicing with moderation. Tai chi is one of the few disciplines where the more you strain, the less you gain. Tai chi rewards the intelligent under-achiever, not the super-achiever

- Many people take tai chi courses from the same person over and over again, because each time they learn to refine and benefit more from the same physical movements. As their external movements and coordination improve, they focus less on external movements and more on the internal ones

- Many students focus on learning movements correctly or doing them "perfectly." They ask, "Am I doing this move correctly?" What they should ask is, "Am I improving?" or "How can I do this move better?" As some advanced students say, "The first ten years is only a warm-up."

Although tai chi is not especially easy to learn, it is not the most difficult thing to do either. Half of China's 200 million people who successfully learned and currently do tai chi every day began after age fifty. If they can learn, you can.

Some degree of challenge makes most recreational activities more fun, interesting, and alive, whether they are physical (golf, skiing, tai chi), mental (reading good books, doing crossword puzzles), or artistic (playing music, painting). Lack of any challenge causes many activities to become boring, causing people to quit. Conversely, all worthwhile activities that continue to have both short- and long-term pay-offs usually have continuing challenges.

Tai Chi: Levels of Complexity

As mentioned in Chapter 8, all Taoist practices are based on three treasures that are inherent to human beings: body, energy, and spirit, in Chinese called *jing, chi, shen.* In one view, body is considered tai chi's foundation and energy its advanced practices. If you don't have a spiritual interest, doing only energy and body work will make you able to function more powerfully in practical, day-to-day worldly affairs.

Spirit is considered Taoism's advanced spiritual potential, which rests on the shoulders of body and energy.[1] Working with spirit can release the deeper stresses and bring about the emotional transformations that make your mind and body fully conscious, opening and deepening spiritual awareness.

The three treasures can be thought of as a continuum: energy work supercharges body work, and spirit work supercharges energy work; body work supercharges energy work, and so on. So even though advanced practices exist, all practitioners must begin at and always return to the level of the body. Within the entire tradition, body, spirit, and energy have their own distinct spheres of direct influence. Each also includes some aspects and techniques intimately

---

[1] Chinese medicine and Taoist meditation have a different perspective on what *shen* or spirit is. Any teacher of tai chi may view this subject from either camp or mix and match the two, depending upon the context of what they are teaching.

interconnected to and mixed with the others. This makes in effect nine potential areas of emphasis: for example energy (or spirit) aspects related to the body, or the body and energy aspects of spirit, etc.

Body

The physical body is the container through which your energy and spirit flow. This is the physical approach to health, longevity, and optimum performance. Through tai chi you learn how to exercise the body down to its most subtle aspects. This can best be done if you understand the body's physical mechanisms and realities, such as anatomical subtleties or how different parts of the body do or don't work well and flow together.

Most tai chi students and teachers begin with the level of body. As the student progresses, the relevant energetic and spirit techniques which are directly related and germane to actualizing the potentials of the body will be brought in.

Energy

The legendary martial arts abilities of many tai chi masters derive from the development of the many functional kinds of subtle chi-energy. This is where many of the "secrets" are hidden in tai chi and for which some train arduously over decades to achieve and master. This energy level of tai chi is also what produces its powerful capacity to heal. The energy level is a potential gateway to human intuitive or psychic capacities. It also can enable overly energetically sensitive or psychically developed individuals to ground and smooth their energy, so they can handle—rather than be overwhelmed—by their natural inner capabilities. Some tai chi masters or instructors work with chi development but don't like to call it as such, for various reasons. Many are unable to explain its mechanisms clearly. Others talk about chi a lot, but can't "walk the talk."

Some tai chi students have a natural talent for working with energy; some don't. Some energetically sensitive individuals think they can; but in reality do so only feebly. Some feel chi-energy early on; others not for years or decades, if at all. Others have chi-energy working strongly and growing within them but don't consciously experience it except as ordinary physical experiences that just seem to make their body work better.

Although some forms of chi gung start working with chi-energy purely at the energetic level with minimal physical work, this is not so for tai chi. The foundation of energy level work in tai chi is working the body, *jing*, the physical. Even though your emphasis may be on chi-energy, the physical work of tai chi must be accomplished. Comments like "just feel the energy flow within you" are normally insufficient to develop chi. If chi can be compared to bio-electricity, electricity can be most valuably used if it operates through a well-functioning device: a computer, refrigerator, machine, etc. Students must learn the physical movements and body alignments for tai chi to produce its energetic benefits.

Spirit (Mind)

Spirit's sphere of influence works directly with the mind and the invisible spirit within us. It involves the arts and sciences of meditation, which originally generated the first two levels of body and energy. Spirit involves active use of the mind. It tells your body and chi-energy when and how to move. Using your spirit well is mandatory to fully engage your capacity to get to the roots of true personal power, obtain emotional balance and inner peace, and actualize the potential of the mind. While intent can take you a long way with body and energy, the heart-mind is required to fully activate spirit. The heart-mind is the center of your consciousness, the place where thoughts and images come from before they reach the conscious level.

Working with body, energy, and spirit has within it beginning, intermediate, and advanced techniques. They are learned much the same way as music: basic techniques build on each other until you can seamlessly blend them. The art of tai chi is as complex as the greatest symphony. At its most advanced stages the body, mind, and spiritual components blend into a unified whole that lead you to experiencing the Tao. Unlike learning music, however, where you progress by learning successively more challenging pieces of music, in tai chi you perform the same series of movements, each time going deeper and learning more.

What You Can Expect to Learn

In tai chi, who is the beginner? This is truly a trick question. Even after twenty years of practice, many students genuinely consider themselves beginners, especially after watching a high level tai chi master at work.

Tai chi's beginning, intermediate, and advanced practices are like a continuum without exact defining landmarks. Criteria and standards of what constitute beginning, intermediate, or advanced methods vary widely between individual teachers and entire schools of tai chi. Some teachers have a larger, more complete knowledge of the entire tradition than others. Consequently, one group's idea of what constitutes an advanced technique, by another group's standards may be considered something only marginally more advanced than the basic level.

For this book's purpose, a beginner is defined as someone who is interested in, experimenting with, and still deciding if they want to commit to tai chi. This means they have taken classes or done tai chi for a year or less.[2]

Within these classes you can expect to learn:

- sequences of movements
- basic body alignments
- the 70 percent rule (moderation)
- coordination
- how to protect your joints.

You may also be taught a few of the components of the nei gung system (see p. 226), that extends into and through tai chi's more advanced energy work.

During the first year, unless you are exceptionally sensitive, it is unreasonable to expect to feel a lot of chi. Although at its advanced levels, tai chi's primary goal is to grow and balance your chi, for the beginner, thinking about these exercises only from the perspective of chi-energy is neither necessary nor desirable. Staying grounded in the body tends to keep any self-perceived experiences of energy from being overly exaggerated or pure fantasy.

Tai chi's physical movements work as effective sensitivity and awareness exercises, which keep the body flexible, reduce stress, and tone and strengthen muscles. For health and longevity, you practice tai chi as non-impact physical exercise and ignore the idea of energy.

Learning to Practice with Moderation: the 70 Percent Rule

Tai chi's greatest challenge for Westerners is learning the timeless art of moderation—neither doing too much nor too little—or the 70 percent rule. The core of the 70 percent rule says you should use your full effort and energy, but not to the point of strain. It advocates maintaining a natural comfort zone rather than using force to push your limits. If this is done, it allows you to easily absorb and integrate inside yourself the fruits of your efforts and to build on them without resistance to practicing again the next day.

The 70 percent rule also helps prevent injuries when learning tai chi. From the very beginning, a good teacher will tell you not to bend and overextend your knees past your toes, because it will put weight and strain on them and could eventually cause problems with the knee joints.

---

[2] In classic tai chi, most students were considered beginners for the first 10 years, intermediate students for the next 10, and only would be deemed advanced students after 20 to 30 years.

Strain on the joints is commonly experienced as a burning sensation.

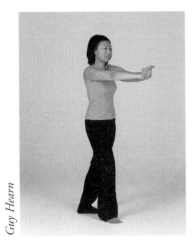

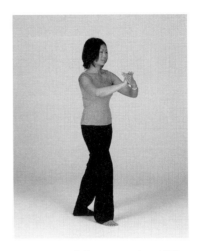

Guy Hearn

The tai chi move Press Forward *done incorrectly at 100% extension, with locked elbows and raised shoulders*

Press Forward *done correctly at 70% extension, with bent elbows and dropped shoulders*

The 70 percent rule applies to everything you learn and do in tai chi—whether it be physical, mental, energetic, or spiritual. It is explored more fully in Chapters 3 and 4.

Important considerations for a beginner in applying the 70 percent rule:

Movement	Only extend or retract arms or legs to 70 percent of their potential range of movement, so you never fully lock them. This prevents joint damage and increases the fluid pumping capacity of the joints (see p. 53 in Chapter 3). Only do stances 70 percent as low as your legs, hips, and spine can handle. Only turn your hips and waist 70 percent as far as they can go to the left or right.
Practice	Only practice 70 percent as long as your physical stamina lasts.

Because it is normal to do the movements without strain, but still feel the muscles ache, a routinely asked question is, "How am I supposed to relax when my muscles feel strained?" This stage of effort must be engaged in before the stage of non-effort can be achieved. The ultimate goal of tai chi is to have your muscles experience little or no strain, but that is more the way of an intermediate or advanced student, not one who is just beginning. Staying within the 70 percent rule will help get you there.

Body Alignments

Fundamental to all forms of tai chi (and chi gung and other Taoist martial arts) are body alignments, from the gross to the subtle. (See Chapter 3, p. 55.)

The Basic Tai Chi Posture

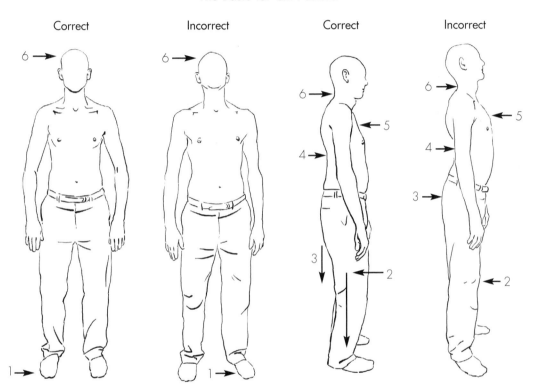

Correct   Incorrect   Correct   Incorrect

Correct Alignments

1. Feet parallel, shoulder-width apart
2. Knees slightly bent and center of knee over center of foot
3. Pelvis slightly tucked under, tailbone perpendicular to the ground
4. Spine gently straightened
5. Chest slightly rounded and dropped without collapsing
6. Head and neck straight, eyes and nose parallel to floor

Incorrect Alignments

1. Feet not parallel
2. Knees locked and not over center of foot
3. Buttocks and tailbone protruding backwards
4. Back not straight, excessively arched
5. Chest pushed out and raised
6. Head tilting backwards

Few adults have perfect body alignments: over time their ankles may have collapsed, their spine might become twisted, their midriff shrunk, one shoulder may be higher than the other, the neck may be a little crooked, etc. The purpose of learning body alignments is that they enhance the circulation of all the bodily fluids and chi. Tai chi gradually teaches you to take the kinks out of your body, making you healthier, stronger, and able to release whatever energies are bound within you.

Your instructors are likely to teach you the basic tai chi posture—feet parallel, shoulder-width apart, knees centered over the feet, tailbone pointed to the ground, spine gently straightened, chest rounded and slightly sunk, and head and neck straight and perpendicular to the ground. You will be encouraged *not* to bend your knees so that they extend past your toes, to prevent excess strain and eventual injury. Good body alignments ensure that you do not put excess pressure on and harm the knees. The knees are not designed to bear the weight of your body; instead they are supposed to act as a conduit to transfer your weight through them to the ground.[3]

Correct Knee Alignment for Forward Weighted Stance

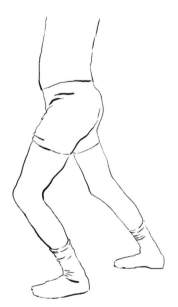 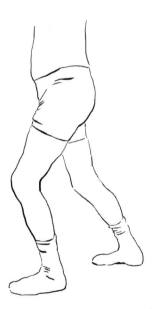 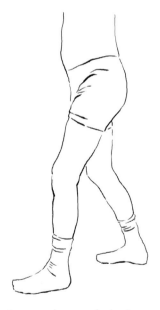

Incorrect: knee too far forward, beyond toes	*Correct: center of knee directly over center of foot, not beyond toes*	*Incorrect: knee too far back, center of knee at or behind heel*

---

[3] Correct knee alignments are discussed in detail in my book, *Opening the Energy Gates of Your Body* (North Atlantic Books, 1993), pp. 86–90.

Learning Tai Chi Sequences

Learning the external movement sequences of tai chi follows the same relative structure as learning how to write in most languages. There are five basic stages.

1. **Letters of an alphabet.** First you learn the different pieces of any individual tai chi movement—what your hands, arms, waist, legs, and feet do independently and in coordination with each other

2. **String the letters into comprehensible whole words.** You learn to combine small individual movements into a single, coordinated movement, in tai chi commonly called a posture, such as *Brush Knee* or *Play the Lute*

3. **Create phrases and sentences.** You learn how a series of movements (postures) becomes connected by a common theme, either in terms of physical or energetic goals. For example, in the Yang and Wu styles the most well known of these series is composed of five movements with the poetic name of *Grasp Sparrow's Tail*

4. **You make longer and longer sentences.** You learn to make longer sequences that conclude in a single posture, such as *Single Whip* (especially in the Yang and Wu styles)

5. **Make paragraphs.** When learning the long forms, you string many connected sentences together until each becomes a paragraph unto itself. In the Yang and Wu styles, for example, the long forms are usually divided into three "paragraphs," which are called sections.

Whatever specific style you do, your efforts will first be directed toward trying to accurately mimic the shape of each individual movement and remember sequences. At first, you will learn where to place your hands and feet, when to shift weight and what direction to turn in. Learning the correct directions challenges the memory and is tricky for many. Long forms usually require you to alternately face in or move in eight directions, based on the eight points of a compass; short forms usually require you to work only with four or six directions.

Most of the time you will be moving. Some teachers, however, may ask you to hold the end point of a single moving posture for a few minutes at a time in order to stabilize its qualities within you and show you the correct alignments for each posture. At first your main focus is to learn the individual movements (postures) and the transitions between them, which for many can be as complex as the original movements. Later, you will learn to improve the outer movement qualities of the postures, and later still, especially if you are an intermediate student, work with the invisible internal qualities of the postures.

For beginners who are primarily interested in health and longevity practices, particularly in the West, it is less common to learn individual postures first, stand for a while in the posture, and then learn the moving transitions between them. In the Yang and Wu styles this was a classical method commonly used when teaching tai chi with a strong martial arts emphasis. It is equally uncommon for beginners to learn tai chi sitting practices.

Month by month, you will progressively experience the same moves differently, not only because you are absorbing what you heard the first time around, but more importantly, because the moves are opening up your ability to feel your body, and possibly your chi.

Coordination

Tai chi gives a completely new meaning to the idea of whole-body coordination. Over time it will increase this, whether or not you are naturally gifted with physical coordination.

The first challenge is to coordinate the left and right sides of your body, for example, the movement of the left arm with the right leg so that both move at the same relative speed. For virtually everyone, one side of the body is stiffer, number, weaker, or more unresponsive than the other. This is normal. Most people are surprised about this. Only a fraction of the population is symmetrical, with the right and left sides fully balanced.

The second coordination challenge occurs when you try to get your hands to move smoothly along with the rest of your arm, rather than stubbornly by themselves.

The third challenge will be to have the waist and arms move together, or the waist and feet, which befuddles most beginners and makes them realize how much looser their hips could be. Even experienced martial artists or dancers, who are supposed to be beyond this, find that it is difficult to get their arms and legs to move in smooth coordination with their waist. Everyone goes through this problem.

However, if you accept these challenges, over time you will also strongly increase your general level of physical coordination. This opinion is derived from repeated observation of many thousands of tai chi practitioners who gain a high degree of coordination, whether they were totally inactive couch potatoes, uncoordinated types, or highly active and skilled athletes. Tai chi will also empower your self-image by showing you what your body is capable of doing.

In this respect it is useful for younger people to remember that half of China's 200 million or more daily practitioners begin tai chi after age fifty. At this stage of life, although the ease of acquiring higher levels of physical coordination is not at a natural high point, most are able to learn tai chi.

Protecting Your Joints

Because tai chi movements thoroughly work the joints, special care must be taken not to injure them. Aside from respecting the 70 percent rule, you will be taught *never to lock* any joint by straightening it during any movement. A clear sign that tai chi teachers have not been properly trained is if they omit this very important principle.

From a health and longevity standpoint, locking a joint cuts off the circulation of fluids; from a martial arts standpoint, locked joints are extreme points of vulnerability because they can be so easily snapped or dislocated by an opponent. Many people understand that during falls and car accidents, breakages commonly occur at the joints because people instinctively lock them. Holding the steering wheel with locked elbows can make whiplash a lot worse, because the shock wave goes more forcefully into your neck and spine.

Although tai chi does not specifically train falling techniques as is common in many martial arts, an often-told story is that when a tai chi practitioner does take an unexpected tumble, it seems to occur in such slow motion that they remember not to lock their joints and therefore do not break or dislocate them, as commonly happens for many. The regular practice of tai chi helps you gain awareness of relaxing your joints in all circumstances.

You will also be taught to be aware of a major warning sign that occurs if you do overwork your joints: a burning sensation or any other kind of pain *inside the joints* are major warning signs that you are most likely overworking them. If this happens, you must back off whatever in your practice is making it occur. Muscles can burn and ache without long-term damage, but not joints.

Challenges that Beginners Normally Encounter

It is natural to repeatedly forget how to do individual moves or which direction to face. Either learning or doing, everyone initially finds some moves more difficult than others. Do not feel discouraged if you sometimes remember and sometimes forget what move comes before or after another. It happens to everyone. Sooner or later, the order more or less sticks in your mind, and you no longer need to follow someone to keep up.

The traditional way to remember movements would be for a teacher to show how specific postures could be used for self-defense. Even if you are not interested in tai chi as a martial art, seeing the self-defense applications of moves makes them easier to remember.

Weight-shifting movements and kicking sequences may challenge your balance and the stretching ability of your legs. Almost universally, beginners find it difficult to keep their shoulders down and their knees from not excessively bending or locking. Perhaps your joints lack flexibility or your hips may be tight or injured, which makes squatting low difficult for you.

Until your leg muscles strengthen, it is quite common for them to ache after doing the movements continuously for more than ten minutes. Although tai chi *looks easy*, especially in the beginning, *it is not*. Expect to work hard and get some sore muscles, but remember the 70 percent rule to protect your joints. For many there is a mental disconnection between how effortless tai chi looks and how difficult the movements are to learn. It befuddles most that the seemingly simple movements fully engage all you have to put out.

At either obvious or subliminal levels, the boundary line between exercised and strained muscles is where your soft tissues feel like tight wires ready to snap. This is the point to pull back so that you do not pull your anatomical tissues out of alignment without your knowing (due to a lack of body sensitivity) and destabilize or injure them. As with sport, the pain and dysfunction of overstrain may occur hours or days after the time of injury. You need to learn to apply moderation before it happens.

Expect the movements, in many subtle ways, to make you realize just how much you lack coordination. This is a shock to many, particularly highly skilled athletes, dancers, and other movement specialists. It is very common for many to find that the coordination required to do the movements well is an unexpected challenge.

The Challenges of Learning Large and Small Frame Tai Chi Styles

Feng Zhi Qiang of Beijing, one of China's most important Chen style masters, has said that the defining characteristic of a tai chi style is not so much what style it is but whether it uses large, medium or small frame movements.

During the early phases of learning, there are trade-offs to be considered when choosing a large or small frame style. However, at the end of the day, all styles will get you to the same place.

There is a continuum between large and small frame styles. At one end of the spectrum, there is the absolute large frame with its stretched-out arm movements and low stances and no small movements. At the other extreme are incredibly tiny movements, high stances, and no dramatic extensions of the arms. Both the Yang (large frame) and the Wu (small frame) will begin with relatively large movements and make them smaller over time as a person advances. The difference between large and small frame styles is how large or small their movements will end up being.

With a larger frame style, expect your leg muscles, especially the thighs, to ache. This is due to the longer stances, and is most noticeable when shifting all your weight to your back leg.

With a small frame style expect the strain on your legs and knee joints to be less because of their generally higher and shorter stances. Small frame styles are ideal for people who are overweight or have weak or injured lower backs and knees.

Large frame movements work and stretch the body's larger, more visible muscles, such as those of the calf, waist, shoulders, and back, and can strain the knees and lower back more.

Although smaller frame styles also work the big muscles, they do not do it as much as the large frame styles. However, small frame styles stretch the body's deeper layers of fasciae, tiny ligaments, etc., more, especially those just next to the spine and neck, around the internal organs, joints (with the shoulder blades being particularly noticeable), and deep within the pelvis. Because smaller circular movements somewhat bypass the larger soft tissues, the pulling and stretching actions target areas deeper inside the body, such as the insertion points of your soft tissues, and your internal organs, more than the long muscles themselves.

Larger circular movements require somewhat less physical coordination than small frame movements, and physically are relatively easier to do. However, in small frame styles, the trade-off becomes that a little more difficulty in physical coordination gives you greater access and a greater ability to work with your chi-energy and more positively affect the body's deeper layers, especially the internal organs. Small frame movements demand more energetic sensitivity initially; however, over time they allow you to get control of your chi in a more direct manner.

Breathing

For at least your first year of tai chi, it is best to begin with natural breathing. You simply inhale and exhale in the way that is most comfortable to you at any given moment, and do not try to coordinate inhales and exhales with specific movements.

There are four main reasons for doing this:

- It gives you the time to sort out and consciously recognize the felt qualities of your deeper subliminal and overt emotional tensions. With experience, you begin to find inner awareness tools that empower you to consciously relax, and reduce or completely neutralize your negative emotions
- It tells you how far you can push your internal subliminal emotional waters before suffering a backlash
- It gently establishes healthy relaxation rhythms, which prevent hidden stress responses from taking hold
- It enables your nervous system to more easily adjust to all the new neurological input and changes the movements are creating within you, thereby making physical relaxation easier.

Breathing naturally allows your physiology to find its own base level, before adding the complications of specific breathing rhythms to modulate the ratio between inhales and exhales in coordination with the movements in a tai chi form.

Natural breathing helps you avoid unleashing suppressed emotions too quickly and explosively. Breath affects the chi. From the perspective of chi-energy, the thoughts and emotions moving through us are also composed of waves of chi. The combination of movement and breath not only controls your physical chi, it also can activate your suppressed emotions.

Trying to control your breath too soon can easily render you incapable of feeling, recognizing, or relaxing these suppressed volcanoes stirring inside, which you might unconsciously energize before pushing them down and controlling them yet more. After tai chi practice is over, without consciously knowing what is going on or why, these energized suppressions can reemerge and explode, for example as anger, fear, or depression.

Learning Strategies for Beginners

Anything subtle like tai chi takes a little time before what it is can be recognized and appreciated, and you can get its potential benefits. Tai chi has great depth and is learned over time, even by the most talented people. Even though you can learn the basic movements of a short form in a week-long retreat, it takes time for the movements to work deeply into your body and for you to feel how tai chi is changing you.

This long-range approach runs counter to that of those people who are cruising spiritual supermarkets, sampling this or that philosophy, exercise, diet, meditation, etc. Although this approach provides entertainment value and alleviates life's boredoms, it rarely satisfies deeper needs. As an old spiritual saying goes, "In a really dry place you have a better chance of finding sweet water by drilling a hole two hundred feet deep, than ten holes twenty feet deep." If you want to discover if tai chi suits you and allows you to hit satisfying, long-term pay dirt, you must stay with it a good while, possibly for years.

This is what works best:

- Unless you are incredibly self-disciplined, you need regular weekly classes to establish energetic rhythms within your body and central nervous system. Without these rhythms many Westerners find it nearly impossible to get into the regular habit of doing tai chi. Modern society fights being regular at anything except earning a living: everything else seems to take a back seat. Although tai chi is something that can help keep you healthy and unstressed, regularity is essential to achieve this. As you begin to establish regular rhythms and schedules, you will be able to consistently practice tai chi daily without needing the reinforcement of regular weekly classes

- The easiest path to regular practice is sticking with one form. By all means, shop around for which form you want to do, but then settle and stick with it

- Learn the basics thoroughly. If you lack these, the most valuable tai chi benefits will not come to you, no matter how many years you practice. That is why it is best to have regular contact with a teacher to help correct your movements and alignments, and help you progress in your learning

- What if you feel that your teacher can't help you progress? If after investigation, you find another local teacher who can do the job much better and decide to change teachers, it is good to do so before bad habits become ingrained. Even if the change involves learning a different style or form, now that your body has the energetic rhythm of doing tai chi, the long-term benefits of getting better basics will far outweigh the extra effort of having to learn new movements

- If no adequate teacher is available locally, the next best solution is to attend trainings of reputable teachers and masters in other locations to get exposed to quality basics. You then take the knowledge home and integrate it into your form as best you can

- Above and beyond solid basics, there exists tai chi's more advanced material. At this point it may be useful to attend other masters' workshops to understand the potentials and see if they appeal to you. A potential side benefit of this might be that this will help you gain insight into what your local teacher may obviously know and do, but may not be able to communicate effectively.

Practice Strategies for Beginners

When first learning tai chi, if you have an over-scheduled life and just want to take care of everyday physical discomforts with the least amount of effort, a more easy-going practice schedule is better and more realistic than training full-bore with a perfectionist attitude. Initially trying too hard usually creates significantly more tension than trying too little. You want to shift out of the habit of creating stress. Rather, take it easy and use tai chi's slow-motion movements as a retraining process to relax and pace yourself to avoid the cumulative stress damage that can result from trying too hard.

A softer approach will better help to promote chi circulation.

Ideally, do some tai chi at a regular time each day, either by yourself or with a group, even if only for a short time, such as five minutes. You can do it for longer periods to extend your regular practice or at other times during the day, but setting a regular practice time for the first ten years, even if only for five minutes, will make a tremendous difference in your long-term progress. Practicing regularly will benefit you more than not doing any tai chi during the week and trying to make up for it by doing long sessions on the weekends.

The best time to practice is sometime, rather than no time at all. Only a few minutes of tai chi every day allows your nervous system to keep continuity with relaxation and to not forget how to consciously get chi to flow. By keeping a regular rhythm, you will most likely find yourself effortlessly extending your practice, in a way that fits your lifestyle of ever changing moments. This said, there is another way to look at this question.

From a purely physical point of view, it takes the body about twenty minutes of continuous exercise for blood to fully engorge the blood vessels enough to make a significant difference. This is a necessary requirement for enabling any kind of cardiovascular exercise (including tai chi, walking, or running) to provide benefits. From this perspective, doing tai chi for twenty minutes at a time, four or five days a week, is quite sufficient to achieve basic health benefits.

To enter the middle ground between health and true fitness, simply increase the total cumulative time you do the form, or add supplementary chi gung exercises.

Conclusion

The teacher leads you to the door of knowledge. However, only through your personal practice can you gain tai chi's profound benefits. To integrate the most profound benefits within your body may take many months or years depending on your focus, intent, goals, natural talent, the quality of your practice, and how much time you spend doing it.

Don't be concerned if you feel that you are not doing specific movements very well. Give yourself time to absorb the big shapes of the movement. The most important thing is to learn the whole sequence together even if you have to fudge some moves. This builds confidence for the long haul. Refining the moves happens with practice, or in the next rounds of learning new information.

If you have specific moves you really like, do them singly outside the sequence of the form. This builds up your confidence and creates the foundational skills needed to eventually overcome the bigger challenges of more difficult moves.

Do not emotionally beat yourself up over moves that you personally find difficult. Just move on and complete the entire sequence as best you can. Don't get hung up on one or two moves. You will improve with practice.

Do not compare your learning speed to others. Tai chi is challenging for everyone to learn.

Above all, be patient with yourself.

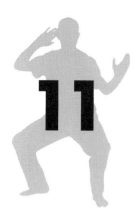

11

Intermediate and Advanced Students:

What You Can Expect to Learn

The intermediate and advanced stages of learning tai chi only begin after you can remember the external movements. By this time your body's alignments have stabilized and your external muscles have relaxed enough for you to begin to consciously soften and relax deep inside your

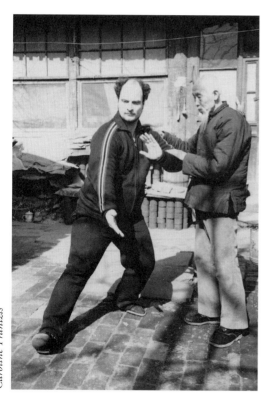

Caroline Frantzis

The author begins the Wu style Shoulder Stroke movement while being corrected by Liu Hung Chieh in his Beijing Courtyard

body. Then you can begin to focus on tai chi's internal movements, breathing, more sophisticated coordination, and chi development. Many students and teachers do not have enough clarity or experience to always know whether a given technique is advanced or not. Many teachers learn advanced material from a higher-level master and then almost immediately (before they have truly assimilated the information) teach it inappropriately to relatively new students. Although this makes it more interesting for the teacher's learning process (and often intellectually fascinating for the student), it usually confuses and does the beginning student a disservice. It is incumbent upon both students and junior teachers to adhere to a master's words regarding when, where, and how each specific more advanced technique can be usefully implemented.

For sincere students it is good advice to

go step-by-step and drop the desire to skip ahead, if you ultimately want your practice to bear maximum fruit.

The Greater the Challenge, the Greater the Rewards

One of my Yang style teachers, T.T. Liang, was a wonderful example of overcoming continuous challenges and refusing to be scared off by tai chi's hidden complexities. Liang began tai chi when he was around fifty because he had severe health problems caused by a life of dissipation (alcohol, opium, and gambling addictions) in pre-Communist Shanghai.

After tai chi helped him restore his health, he focused on the next challenge: becoming a skilled tai chi fighter. After twenty years, his chi became strong enough to effectively fight against strong and highly skilled martial artists in their prime. His perseverance enabled him to delve deeply enough into advanced tai chi practices to become a genuine tai chi master.

During the last thirty years of his life, he lived and taught in America. He credited the continuous practice of tai chi with enabling him to live until he was over a hundred years old.

Integrating the Three Treasures

Intermediate and advanced practices increasingly incorporate and integrate the three treasures of body, energy, and spirit into everything you do in tai chi.

Body

More sophisticated body practices:

- implement tai chi's most minute super-alignments
- move internal organs in coordination with the tai chi postures
- internally stretch the body's deepest substructures
- fully use the springiness of the ligaments
- apply Taoist breathing techniques
- revolve primarily around physical movements, as in the beginning practices, with some standing methods and occasionally sitting ones
- emphasize circularity of movement
- incorporate twisting and spiraling.

Energy

At intermediate and advanced stages, students are introduced to all the possibilities of how chi-energy works.

The fullness of this level of tai chi is generally only known or taught by martial tai chi masters. Push hands, traditional weapons, and all tai chi's martial arts skills are usually the medium by which the overwhelming majority of genuine masters teach tai chi's complete chi-energy methods.

Here is where the specific details and aspects of all 16 nei gung components are taught. Mastering them is crucial to obtaining success in the highest worldly possibilities tai chi has to offer, such as health, stress relief, longevity, or developing tremendous high-performance physical skills and internal power.

Standing postures and sitting techniques may be used extensively at this stage of practice.

Spirit

All the possibilities of how spirit work is imparted, using Taoist methods, to create spiritual evolution that culminates in what some called enlightenment. When tai chi rises to this level of practice it becomes what this book refers to as Taoist tai chi. (See Chapter 8, p. 151.) Taoist tai chi's way to engage in this level requires the foundation of both body and energy. No matter how rarified work with spirit or energy becomes, simultaneously in tai chi there is always a concrete, ongoing awareness of the body. Then through the mind you contact and explore the possibilities of spirit. Even in China those who can teach this level of tai chi at the more advanced levels are rare. Standing practices are done relatively little; instead practices primarily alternate between moving and sitting.

All Taoist practices are based on achieving balance at all levels of the human condition: physical, emotional, mental, psychic, and spiritual. Having yin-yang relationships function with maximum efficiency is the centerpiece of tai chi body and energy practices.

However, to Taoists, true balance requires the capacity to live freely and function well, from a place that concurrently transcends and is the source of all yin-yang relationships. This is a quiet yet vibrant, non-dual space that is permanent and unchanging amid all yin-yang variations and is the necessary breeding ground from which true universal love and compassion can grow. This is a central point and goal of spirit practices. This non-dual transcendence is what the philosophical term *tai chi* literally means in Chinese.

Along the path, developing spirit means:

- releasing your inner demons (disturbed emotions), either by transforming or dissolving them
- establishing positive emotions
- reducing overall emotional negativity
- restoring physical, emotional, and spiritual balance
- getting in touch with your psychic potential.

To achieve this requires learning internal techniques, either solo or with practice partners, which will help you to:

- work with organs and glands
- come into harmony with the forces of nature
- work with the esoteric energies of the five elements, and the environment including the sun, moon, planets, and stars
- use all three tantiens (see pp. 230–231), not only the lower one, which is sufficient for body and energy work
- work with your left, right, and central energy channels.

More About the 70 Percent Rule for Experienced Students

Adhering to the 70 percent rule can save you years of relatively unproductive effort in reaching the relatively more advanced stages of tai chi. This holds true whether your interest is optimum health, high performance in martial arts or athletics, or intellectual achievement. Without adhering to the 70 percent rule, it is difficult to reach the most profound depths of spirit, because going for 100 or 150 percent makes it difficult to let go of the ego.

Range of Motion   If you are in great shape, and intimately know your limits to a razor's edge, you may go a little over 80 percent of your physical range of motion limits. This, however, not 90 percent, is the absolute upper range. This is especially true for tai chi's twisting and spiraling techniques and its deeper internal stretches.

Practice Time	Only practicing 70 to 80 percent as long as your physical and energetic stamina can last.
Chi-energy	Only putting out or absorbing 70 percent as much chi as you feel capable of.
Spirituality	Consciously attempting to stay in any spontaneous spiritual expansion or altered state only while it is easy to maintain it effortlessly; that is, without attempting to use mental force to maintain or extend the duration of the experience.

The Transition from External to Internal Movements

As your external movements become more coordinated and fluid, you will gradually, and often randomly, begin to get some surprising internal sensations. A door opens to feeling your insides. You begin to become aware of the pulls and stretches at the points of connection (insertion points) where muscles, ligaments, tendons, and bones meet. Or you begin to feel something inside the center of your joints, rather than only the muscles that surround them. Or you might feel the inside of your belly and some of your internal organs.

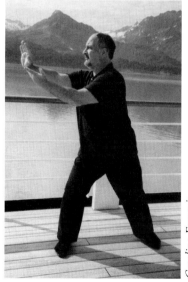

Wu style Cloud Hands. *This quintessential movement incorporates almost all the core principles of tai chi in the Yang and Wu styles*

Caroline Frantzis

Perhaps you experience intermittent flashes of energy inside your body—points on your hands or feet that light up with tingles of electricity. Or you feel something going up your spine, or a burst of energy from your spine through your arms to your fingertips.

Maybe you begin to experience your lower tantien, first as a vague feeling, then like a reservoir filled with a surprising something, and still later with vibrant pulsation or the still depths of a great ocean.

You now experience how the outer, external movements have the potential to take you deep inside your body and mind. The awakening to your internal energy possibilities within has begun. In tai chi this process is called "from the outside in," or "from external to internal."

Internal Movements

Now you begin to move into the stage of practice where deliberate actions deep inside your body create and generate each external movement. You move from the inside out. Previously, your thoughts focused on how the muscles of your limbs and waist should move, then feeling your body, and next activating your arm muscles to get your hand to move from, say, your hip upwards to well out in front of your body.

Progressively, your awareness now focuses on different invisible places inside your body. These spots then generate the fundamental impulses to move the muscles of your hand or waist. The progression might move from stretching the insertion points of various muscles, to activating specific energy channels, to expanding the fluids inside your joints, or any of the other internal techniques contained within the Taoist 16-part nei gung system (see p. 226). With increasing awareness, familiarity, and experience, you begin to consciously understand how moving and affecting the deep insides of your body can create your external movements. In tai chi this is called "the inner moves the outer." Gradually, the mental and energetic abilities necessary to support your inner journey through tai chi are put in place.

Whereas external movements are obvious, internal movements are invisible, yet no less real. Many senior tai chi students and masters have a mysterious aura of chi about them as they practice. This often creates a very positive feeling in the observer. Internal movements create this indefinable something you know is there but can't see.

External and Internal Stretching

Cats stretch incessantly. Their bodies unwind like ripples in water. As they do so, every tiny muscle, each in its own time, stretches and relaxes.

To really advance in your practice, it is important that, like a cat, you neither be self-conscious nor make a big deal that you are stretching either very big or very subtle parts of yourself. Stretching is natural.

Likewise, tai chi movements will release and stretch your body's soft tissues as if you were a cat. In the animal kingdom, cats are one of the better combinations of strength, flexibility, and sheer bounce. They relax and let go of their muscles in order to have them operate so efficiently. Feel how soft a house cat is. Watch the softness of its whole body as it expands and contracts to its breathing rhythm. It is a different model from muscular tension, one that tai chi shares.

Tai chi's external and internal stretches, whether they are of a lengthwise or twisting kind, occur through a very common pattern. Initially if you relax even just a little, your awareness will notice some area of muscular tension. By maintaining your awareness on it, the action of noticing it, combined with the movements themselves, will cause the muscle to gradually release by stages to whatever degree your body is willing. As the form progresses it is quite common for your attention to move on and recognize different tense or tight spots, and begin the whole process of relaxation, awareness, and movement anew.

Tai chi has different levels of external and internal stretching. Sheer lack of movement causes muscles to contract and shorten. Moving through tai chi's postures will let you use muscles you never knew you had and begin to gently stretch them. Your arms and legs act like weights that stretch whatever is connected to your spine, which is ultimately everything in your body.

You first notice external stretches in the big shoulder and leg muscles. Most can't believe just how stiff their shoulders have become and how their necks and backs ache. Gradually, as you do tai chi, you find that your neck naturally clicks into place and that it can turn more easily in all directions, even though you have done no neck-turning exercises.

Then, as the muscles in your chest stretch, you find the pulling on your shoulders, neck, and head gently reducing. As the chest stretches downward, you feel your internal organs begin to drop naturally. Next your breath deepens on its own. Breathing becomes more satisfying, and you become more aware of its possibilities when relaxed.

Shifting weight back and forth while turning the hips can make your legs feel incredibly tired. Yet in time, and in a seemingly miraculous manner, you suddenly find your flexibility and range of motion has dramatically increased. The insides of your body begin to open up. The joints become more supple. Internal stretches pull on all the soft and connective tissues around your joints. When this happens joints can start to naturally pop of their own accord—usually a healthy sign of releasing deep tension. These pops usually begin in the shoulders and hip sockets first. Afterwards they can spread to every joint you have. These pops can be the precursors to your joints regaining the smoothness and flexibility of childhood. However, you should never try to pop your joints forcefully.

At some point the fasciae will begin to stretch. Fasciae are the connective tissues that bind your muscles together so they can function without being overly tight, slack, or floppy. If fasciae become bound, they do not allow your muscles to have free movement, and can create a negative cascading effect where each muscle can bind and diminish other muscles or other anatomical structures from having free movement. Often people's muscles cannot stretch because of the binding of their fasciae.

The bending and stretching movements of tai chi can directly release bound fasciae. This commonly causes sharp pains or burning sensations. The burning discomfort of fasciae stretching does not always feel wonderful, but it is acceptable. However, pain within your joints is not acceptable and usually points to potentially dangerous excess, which indicates an injury in progress. When this begins, it is important to remember the 70 percent rule—go slowly and gently.

These fascia stretches can surprise you. They usually start around the large muscles of the back, neck, and shoulders, and then move to the back, spine, and legs. Finally the fasciae tend to gradually stretch, over months or years, through the chest and into the belly.

After the abdominal muscles relax and open, these fascia stretches then tend to move into the spaces behind your abdominal muscles—the inside of your belly—internal organs, digestive valves, connective ligaments, etc. This process can then release the unnecessary bindings that diminish the workings of the internal organs. This release can help both digestion and elimination immensely. Here again gentleness and keeping to the 70 percent rule is very important. It is definitely best to allow the releases and stretches to come naturally in their own time, rather than attempt to push them along faster.

Inside your body, soft tissues can either stretch towards or away from a point of origin, such as an insertion point. Tai chi movements, in coordination with limbs extending away from, or moving toward, your torso, can accentuate these two kinds of stretching. However, you must first be relaxed enough to recognize the places in your body that are willing to stretch this way, and not try to force the stretch, which will ultimately diminish it.

Stretching towards or away from a tense or bound location in your body usually begins with large external muscles. Over time, as your ability to relax grows, you become able to notice more subtle internal places that are stuck, such as ligaments, membranes, or other anatomical connections within and between your internal organs.

Taoist Breathing

Breath is not chi. However, breath work is a valuable tool through which you can directly contact chi as a felt experience and living reality. The nature of breath in tai chi is that it happens in a peek-a-boo fashion. You notice your breath, then become engrossed in the movements and forget to notice it. It comes, it leaves, it comes, it leaves, until with minimal or no effort you become aware of your breath and your belly all the time.

Regardless of what point you are in the breathing learning curve, it is best to move towards having your breath be long, quiet, soft, relaxed, and continuous without freezing up, shutting down, or stopping.

The breathing process within tai chi and all Taoist breathing methods that allow you to connect with chi go more or less like this[1]:

- Breathe from your nose rather than your mouth. If you are prevented from doing so by congestion, for example colds, flu, sinusitis, or allergies, or by a structural blockage, breathe in and out through the mouth
- Keep your tongue on the roof of your mouth, where the hard palate is located. This is where the tip of your tongue touches when you say "le" in French. This connects two exceptionally important acupuncture meridians, called the governing and conception vessels. Points along these two acupuncture meridians connect to all the yin and yang energies of your body. The place where they meet, where your tongue touches, regulates, and stabilizes the interchange between all the body's yin and yang channels
- Do not hold your breath
- Breathe deeply
- Relax the chest and breathe with the belly. This will strengthen your diaphragm, enabling air to move more efficiently. Do not stick your chest out, or use the front of your chest to breathe
- Use each breath to consciously relax your body. Initially use exhales to focus releasing tension in your physical tissues and nerves. Over time do the same with inhales
- As the belly relaxes, allow the breath to put deeper and deeper pressure on your internal organs
- After you can do all the previous parts comfortably and your nerves have integrated them into your resting breathing in a relaxed, comfortable, and natural fashion, you can gradually add other breathing components, which include:

---

[1] The author's *Longevity Breathing* programs teach these methods.

1. side breathing, which especially benefits the liver and spleen
2. lower back breathing, which especially benefits the kidneys
3. upper back breathing, which uses the back rather than the front of the lungs to breathe. Combined with abdominal breathing, this especially benefits the heart
4. whole back breathing, where all the muscles and other soft tissues that connect with your spine and entire back move in rhythm to your breath
5. spine breathing, at least at more advanced levels. Here, in physical coordination with each breath, all spinal vertebrae come together and separate, while chi-energy moves toward and away, and up and down the spine—a tai chi technique called "the chi sticks to the back."

- Breath goes silent, eyes relax, and although your breath is mechanically doing all the previous steps extremely well and powerfully, the sense of physical air coming in and out of you disappears and everything becomes exceptionally silent inside both your body and mind
- Chi now begins to awaken, and you find yourself experiencing breathing in chi, not air, with each inhale and exhale. This begins the capacity to move and direct your chi purely through your mind. The breath has now lifted the chi airplane off the ground. Although you will still keep the physical mechanics of breathing ongoing, your awareness now shifts from breath to chi
- The link between breath, energy, and consciousness has begun.

Coordinating Movement with Breath

As you become more relaxed, the tendency of your breathing cycle and physical movements to coordinate naturally increases. Your teacher can help you decide whether you are now ready to consciously focus on coordinating your breath with your movements.

This kind of controlled breathing has three extremely beneficial side effects, which is why many intermediate and advanced practitioners prefer it. First, it can unleash a lot of chi, and thereby bestow physical strength and vigor; second, it can make it easier to become accomplished in all tai chi's opening and closing techniques (see p. 231); and third, it can help resolve spiritual blockages. Taoist tai chi uses controlled breathing to gain conscious access to, target, and amplify blocked inner emotional and psychic spaces. It then uses this access to specifically work through, transform, or dissolve these inner blockages.

Some tai chi schools deliberately link breathing and movement, coordinating inhales with the hands moving towards the torso, and exhales with movements away from the torso. Other schools reverse the direction. Both methods can physically create a regular pressure that progressively builds inside your bodily fluids (especially within the abdominal cavity), which, like a steam engine or water pump, can increase pounds of pressure per square inch over time. This generally strengthens the entire body, and specifically the movement of all its internal fluids, conferring health, strength, and vitality. The methods to apply these various breathing techniques or the reasons for teaching one way or another are beyond the scope of this book.[2]

Coordinating breathing with movements too soon can be a double-edged sword. Often this brings up negative emotions faster than an individual's nervous system can handle. Even though it can make the practitioner feel strong, if there are serious hidden demons in the recesses of the psyche, some people may become emotionally unstable.

Health and longevity require an emotional awareness, some level of inner peace and the ability to move chi. Coordinating breath with movement too soon can impede the achievement of these benefits. A good teacher is essential to help you in this process.

Circularity

All tai chi motions involving body, energy, or spirit practices are based on circular movement. The underlying quality of all circles is that they truly have neither a beginning nor an end, just a seamless flowing continuity, where each part of the circle naturally flows into the other unceasingly.

Physically, all hand and foot movements are composed of circles, ellipses, and curving lines, so even something that looks like a straight punch, for example, will have a subtle, gentle arc to it. Energetically, to obtain complete, connected circulation of chi-energy requires you be able to effortlessly establish circles and spirals moving at different speeds within all of tai chi's energetic techniques. The spirit techniques of tai chi also require a circularity of time. Here, the inherent mental, emotional, and psychic tensions contained within the perceptions of past, present, and future flow into a circle with a sense of time and reality that is beyond all three. Nevertheless, you are still pragmatically aware of and able to use the concepts of past, present, and future in daily life.

To get a more concrete sense of circularity, the Chen style of tai chi has a phrase that, loosely translated, says, "the body has eighteen circles," all of which must be separately activated

---

[2] These methods are included in the author's chi gung programs.

and simultaneously combined together. As a whole they create tai chi's physical quality of circularity. These circles may be done in a large, medium, or small frame way. The eighteen are circles made by the:

- **Upper body**: (1) fingers, (2) palms, (3) wrists, (4) elbows, (5) shoulders, (6) shoulder blades and armpits, (7) ribs and sternum, (8) head and neck
- **Mid-body**: (9) waist, (10) spine, (11) internal organs, (12) lower tantien
- **Lower body**: (13) toes, (14) feet, (15) ankles, (16) knees, (17) hip sockets, (18) pelvis and kwa.

Twisting, Spiraling, and Turning

Twisting, turning, and spiraling are some of the most important techniques of tai chi and are integral to all higher-level tai chi capacities, from the gross to the subtle, in terms of health, martial arts, energy, or spiritual work. The primary health benefits of these techniques were discussed in Chapter 3, p. 51. Twisting, turning, and spiraling should be present either in an overt or hidden way within any tai chi technique.

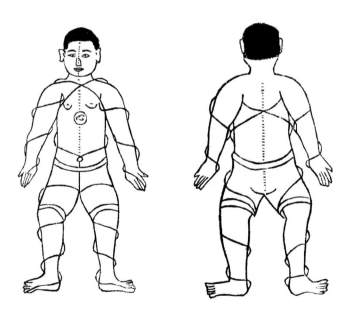

Archival Drawings of the Spiraling of Energy in the Chen Style of Tai Chi

Twisting and spiraling may be the overtly visible, dramatic, and distinguishing characteristic of Chen style tai chi, where it is called spiraling, twisting, or reeling silk. In the most popular tai chi styles (Yang and Wu) twisting and spiraling is more subtle and hidden and is called turning or drilling. Twisting and spiraling continues and amplifies tai chi's fundamental use of circular movements. The joining of multiple circles in a continuous flow creates spirals.

Putting extra work into practicing these twisting and spiraling techniques will maximize the health benefits of tai chi described in Chapter 3. For intermediate and advanced students, there are additional valuable aspects:

- The techniques enhance tai chi's martial aspects by teaching you to efficiently generate power.
  Like high-speed electric power drills, the innate efficiency of turning and spiraling methods create a magnified amount of useable power relative to the energy powering it—especially if compared with generating power by only moving in a straight line, such as when you use a hammer and chisel, or pushing or hitting with your arm or fist.
  When performing yielding techniques in push hands, spiraling methods help you suck in and dissipate your opponent's momentum and power, or redirect their power away from you, while destabilizing their root and center of gravity. When attempting to push your opponent, spiraling methods enable you to have much greater energy discharge power (called *fa jin* in Chinese, and discussed on p. 236). In sparring, they can create powerful strikes and throws, and disguise the origin of your power from opponents, making it more difficult for them to mount an effective defense
- They enhance athletic performance. Spiraling methods will enhance your maneuverability and power. They can increase your ability to project power to hit or throw balls. In swimming, it allows more usable power to be released from your back and shoulders so you can move harder and faster with each stroke. In football, it enables you to withstand strong physical contact better
- They increase the flow of chi through your energy channels. Because chi naturally moves in spirals through the body's energy channels, increasing the spiraling of your physical tissues naturally activates these spirals. This causes energy to move through the channels with greater strength so that you get more chi
- They enhance spiritual practices. Energetic, spiraling movements allow you to directly connect with the energies of heaven and earth, open psychic and intuitive capacities, and have your spirit move beyond being identified with the body.

The Five Progressive Stages

Twisting mimics the process of all previous levels of lengthwise internal stretching and takes them to the next level. The importance of having a competent and thorough instructor to teach these advanced tai chi techniques cannot be overemphasized. The learning process must be taken in five stages slowly, carefully, and gradually, especially when the legs become involved, in order to protect your spine.

1. **Between the fingertips, arms, upper spine, and neck.**

    You will learn to alternately twist between moving toward and then away from the direction of the spine, using all the soft tissues from all parts of your arm, but without twisting the joints themselves. These twists have an amazing ability to release neck and shoulder tension and pain. They also make all the joints of your arm exceptionally flexible within all ranges of movement.

    The process must start in the arms for three reasons:

    a) in most daily activities you consciously use your arms more than other parts of your body, making it relatively easier to feel and comprehend the technique of efficiently twisting. Acquiring this knowledge makes it easier to understand how to do the same for the body parts that most people find more difficult to feel, such as the legs, hips, or internal organs

    b) even with incorrect practice, it is hard to do long-term damage to your arms. Previous life experience has taught most people how to recognize untoward arm pain and strain. Aside from the weight of your own arms there is no massive weight resistance. Consequently it is virtually impossible to tear a rotator cuff as often happens in other physical activities

    c) the upper spine's vertebrae bear less body weight than those of the lower spine. Thus vertebrae there are less likely to go out of place if you twist more than your current limitations will allow (in other words, by forgetting the 70 percent rule). And if they do, they usually give early warning signs with twinges of pain well before they misalign. You thereby gain experience in how to maintain the 70 percent rule and protect your spine. This becomes a vital skill when you later engage the abdominal cavity and lower spine.

2. **Between the toes, legs, and lower spine.**

   Normally significantly harder than twisting the arms, the idea of fully twisting the leg muscles is not a normal idea in Western physical culture. The normal Western lifestyle commonly causes us to have much less feeling in our legs than arms. Reasons abound. In general, the West is an upper body culture where many don't regularly stretch their legs. We wear overly tight shoes that deaden and cut off blood circulation to the feet. We also sit on chairs, and do not tend to squat flatfooted, sit on the ground cross-legged, or walk barefoot.

   The weight of gravity pushes on and will deaden the natural feeling in anyone's legs if something is not done to compensate for the problem.

   You need a competent teacher to teach you twisting in the lower body, and even more so if the twisting is to extend into the internal organs and the soft tissues that affect the entire spine.

   Lower body twisting is a double-edged sword. If done correctly it immensely benefits all the leg joints and spine. However, if done incorrectly it can misalign and harm them. For example, relatively speaking, the knees are structurally the body's weakest joints. Progressively *over-twisting* the knees can result in *long-term damage*, similar to that which can happen within a split second in martial arts when twisting someone's arm with the intent of ripping it apart.

   Equally vulnerable is the lower spine and sacrum. Incorrectly applying twisting techniques or exceeding the 70 percent rule can weaken the ligaments that attach to the lower spine. This can potentially create back pain, by causing the lower back's vertebrae to go out of alignment, the sacrum to become more unstable, and associated back muscles and ligaments to weaken. Given the prevalence of back pain in the West, it is best to learn twisting with a competent instructor

3. **Between the fingertips, neck, chest, and diaphragm.**

   The twisting in the arms extends into the chest, affecting its inner anatomical structures including the lungs and heart. Anatomically the diaphragm connects to and affects all the structures from the arms through the ribs, chest, neck, and head (as well as to the bottom of your pelvis)

4. **Between the toes, hips, and torso to the diaphragm.**

   Initially the twisting begins in the toes, moves up the leg muscles, and then to the external muscles of the buttocks, lower and mid back, sides and front of the waist, and sacrum. Do not deliberately twist the sacrum under any circumstances. In time the twisting, which is generated in the legs, buttocks, and hips can extend through the pelvic floor and progressively enter into and twist the tissues associated with the internal organs within the abdominal cavity, ending in the diaphragm

5. **The twisting and spiraling of your whole body links up.**
    This means that during all tai chi movements, depending on your level of development, there is continuous spiraling:

    a) either towards or away from your body
    b) from your feet to your head or your head to your feet
    c) from the legs, through the abdominal cavity to the head and fingertips, or from the fingertips and head, through the abdominal cavity to the hips, legs, and toes
    d) originating from the lower tantien; the spiral reaches simultaneously to the extremities and returns back again to the lower tantien.

All five of these progressive developmental stages first have a beginning and then an advanced methodology.

Distinctions Between Twisting and Spiraling

The beginning methods of learning *twisting* provide a margin of safety. They loosen your body. As much as possible, these methods ensure that you don't later (in *spiraling*) over-torque and damage your body's weaker areas.

From the perspective of either insertion points or the longer tissues attached to them, you will only twist your soft tissues in one direction at a time. Everything either twists towards your spine, or away from it. These subtle inward and outward twists can also appear to be different depending on whether you initially begin the twisting process with the palm or back of your hand facing you. An instructor is required to make these distinctions clear, as for many they are fairly subtle and counterintuitive.

The *spiraling* method is clearly more advanced. Either moving up or down, the nature of a spiral is not to move only in one direction, but rather it regularly changes its direction from inside to outside as it continues forward on its trajectory. Likewise to spiral the body's inner soft tissues you do the same. For example, the muscles on one part of your arm (legs or waist) go in one direction, and a bit later simultaneously go in the opposite direction. This creates a corkscrew effect that not only works your soft tissues, but coordinates with and results in increased opening and closing of your joints and other structures deep within the abdominal cavity. Again, a competent instructor is absolutely essential to learn this method, as it clearly goes beyond the limits of visible choreography.

Cautionary Notes

The focus of twisting must always begin in the arms, not the legs. It then progresses to the legs through to the pelvis. Only last does twisting focus inside the abdominal cavity. The practitioner must keep to this order. To do otherwise is to indulge in a journey that has the potential to strain or damage your joints and other vulnerable body parts.

Twisting is only done with the body's soft tissues. Never twist within the spine or joints themselves. This can harm you. While soft tissues can twist without harm, harder tissues, such as bone or cartilage, cannot. Twist the soft tissues around the bones, not the bones themselves. If twisted, joints dislocate and tissues tear out of their insertion points, and the joints can potentially develop hairline cracks or worse. For example, if martial artists twist someone's arm *excessively*, and focus the force of the twist into their opponents' muscles it will cause pain, but once released the pain usually quickly dissipates. Conversely, if the force is focused within the joint or the spinal vertebrae they will first dislocate, then crack, and finally break.

Subtle Energy: Chi Development

For most of human history the higher arts of learning how chi-energy works have mostly been kept secret, and only shared with a privileged few. These ancient traditional barriers are beginning to break down, so that access is becoming more openly shared. Nevertheless, the work itself can be definitely challenging. When its components are clearly spelled out, as this chapter attempts, developing chi can sound deceptively easy, in much the same way that golf can sound easy—you just hit a ball through the air and tap it into a hole in the ground. This said, any golfer will tell you that there is much more to the sport than it seems. However, just as many golfers refuse to be put off by golf's hidden complexities, neither should tai chi's advanced chi work scare you off. Just remember, the greater the challenges, the greater the rewards if only you try.

The basic tai chi phrase that describes the process of how human beings can influence their chi from within is called "the mind moves the chi." This occurs in two ways.

The first is through the normal use of awareness, will, and intent. This is the entry point of practice. Here your mind has a specific goal of what you want to occur. You then, without tension, gently focus your will and intent like a laser to accomplish X or Y. This is the way to acquire background, then progressively advance, step-by-step, one stage building on the next, until you reach a high level of chi development.

The second is the heart-mind. This is the center of the energy art of tai chi. In Chinese thought the heart-mind is the center of consciousness in the body, located in the center of the chest next to the physical heart. Here rational intellectual thoughts and what we call the emotional feelings of the heart are one. In the heart-mind, there is no schism between the talking head and heart-felt wisdom. The heart-mind is what makes human beings more than just jumbled emotions or biological thinking machines.

The heart-mind functions before the specific conscious intent to do something arises. The heart-mind merely has a general tendency or possibility. It is diffuse rather than goal-orientated. It flashes with an intelligence that shines before words and intellectual descriptions monopolize your awareness. It also gives your intention the power to function well.

Although intent or will enables you to achieve focused goals, using it exclusively is often myopic and lacking balance. For example, the conscious or unconscious sense of how to achieve your goals often leads either to positive or negative ramifications that can affect your whole being, including the inner and outer environments in which you live. The heart-mind allows you to see the whole forest of consequences; using the intent only allows you to see clumps of trees. It is not at the level of intent, rather it is at the next level of the heart-mind that inner peace, emotional balance, intuition, and spiritual insight arise.

Relatively speaking, intent is the easier way to project your chi in order to do something specific, as well as relax your physical muscles. However, it also can make it harder to relax and release deeper emotional or spiritual tensions that lie below the radar.

Simple and Complex Chi Development

At first, statements about chi usually arrive in very simple sentences: for example, drop your chi to your tantien. On the surface they seem very simple, straightforward instructions. However, after working with these simple instructions, you find that the inner web they open up inside you can become incredibly complex. Felt sensations, emotions, recognition of subtle meanings to all kind of situations your life has led you to, all become part of the fascinating story involved with either, "let this or that happen with your chi," or "have your chi go from here to there." The simple statement takes you through an engaging journey of self-discovery as interesting as seeing major tourist sights of the world, such as the Himalayas or Pyramids. Yet at the end, after all the complexity has surfaced and integrated, it still boils down to the same simple original statement.

Chi is like a mountain you want to climb. On approach it has a simple shape you can recognize and feel comfortable with. However, when climbing it, it ceases to be a mountain. It becomes an infinite series of rocks, paths, handholds, sunny and shady spots, etc. You experience the mountain differently both on the way up and on the way down. Challenging the mountain acts like a focal lens that brings up all sorts of things about your personal life and the ways you perceive, interact, and deal with yourself, people, and events. And yet, once you know the mountain intimately and look at it again, it is still the same mountain. However, now it has a discernable shape more comfortable, interesting, and alive than it appeared on the original approach.

Gross to Subtle

In tai chi, it is said that you only can go as high as your foundation is solid and deep. Developing chi, by its very nature, progresses from the gross (which is easier) to the subtle (which is more difficult). If you have a teacher who is willing and able to teach chi work from the start, it is most useful, even if you can't yet feel the chi-energy inside you, to imagine[3] your chi moving in line with the specific recommendations your teacher gives, so that over time you can develop a sense of it. This can help you benefit even more from the exercises.

How chi works can be intellectually described. However, like love, it has a subtle mysterious quality that must be experienced for it truly to make sense. When encountering the chi of tai chi, it will most reliably happen through a series of basic processes, on which different teachers have different views.

In general, however, the more subtle the chi you are working with in tai chi, the more innate power and capacities it has hidden within, just waiting to be released. Ultimately, however, the maximum benefit occurs when body movements, full intention of the mind, and the movement of the chi all happen together. With gentle patience, over time they will.

Upon recognizing what your own chi feels like, you begin two separate phases that synergistically work with each other. The first is centered on your central nervous system. Having

---

[3] Yang style tai chi teacher T.T. Liang wrote a book that poetically describes this process. It is called *Imagining Becomes Reality* (Dragon Door Publications, 1992).

gained the experience of putting your mind (awareness) into your muscles, you now learn to put it into your nerves. Relaxing and releasing the nerves themselves enables you to recognize the constant nervous buzz that runs through your entire nervous system. Most of us are not aware of this ever-present stressful buzz because it has become so normal. This buzz is a sure sign that your nervous system is either beginning to rev up (like a car going from 0–60 miles per hour in a few seconds), or even worse, has been locked habitually into a constant rev. This rev or buzz is how stress hardens into your body like soft cement into concrete. You now focus on ways to re-soften this nervous buzz inside you, and progressively relax and release it from your nerves.

With a growing capacity to relax, you move into the second phase. Here you want to release the more subtle nervous buzz of blocked chi inside all your body's tissues. Progressively, one by one, you find and release the rev in your joints, blood flow, spinal system, internal organs, and glands. Our modern technological, industrial landscape has created a world that is moving too fast for most to handle. Consequently, it is no surprise that people are becoming ever more numb inside, as a kind of self-defense from being overloaded and overwhelmed. Each stage of releasing the rev from your bodily systems makes your body more awake. This takes you into more subtle and powerful experiences of what it means and feels like for your body to be fully alive. This reawakening can be quite mind-blowing.

An essential part of recognizing and releasing the buzz inside your nervous system is to release any stagnant chi (see p. 59). This may happen naturally as your tai chi improves or because you learn to apply various techniques from the 16-part nei gung system to specifically address stagnant chi issues. Nei gung methods within tai chi that resolve stagnant chi situations include:

- getting the balance right between sinking your chi to the lower tantien and raising chi to the top of the head
- clearing stagnant energy from the left, right, or other channels of the body
- working with various openings and closings (see 16-part nei gung system number 7 p. 230), so that when you are pulsing between opening and closing, you don't get stuck on either end of the pulse.

Resolving stagnant chi conditions can become major ongoing projects.

An Example of One Kind of Progression in Chi Development

Here, technical tai chi terms will be used. Even though you may not understand the meaning of these terms, just try to get the gist of how the general process works for delving deeper into your chi development.

For example, here is what could happen during the journey to actualize the principle of sinking your chi into the lower tantien.

1. The first step requires that you get some part of your intention—your mind or awareness—to stay stabilized in your lower tantien. When that happens, a sense of heat, electricity, fullness, or some other kind of special feeling begins to reside there as a matter of course, without the need to expend much effort to maintain it

2. Progressing to the more subtle, you need to clearly feel chi rising up the spine to the top of your head until that feeling becomes stable

3. Chi must now rise above this point to the energetic boundary of your aura related to your physicality. When this subtle energy becomes stable it draws your spine and head upward, making it relatively easy to maintain space between the spinal vertebrae of your neck. This fulfills the chi principle of "the head is suspended from above as if by a string." The string completes the flow of energy from your physical body to the boundary of your bioelectric body. At this point the sense of chi, although very subtle, becomes concretely felt, as though it is solid matter

4. Going to a yet more subtle level, you must again drop your chi from the top of your head either down your body's front yin acupuncture channels, or down the even more subtle and powerful left, right, or central channels (see the energy anatomy diagrams on p. 228–29). Slowly these very subtle downward flows increase in strength, until a subtle but strong chi flow is continuously felt dropping into your lower tantien during all movements. As each subtle chi flow completes and becomes stable, it kick-starts the next. So as more chi falls, more rises, in a connected, spontaneously repeating circle

5. These rises and falls of energy then set the stage for every point along the ascending and descending energetic pathways to open and pulse in specific rhythms (called "opening and closing" in tai chi, see p. 231). This takes you into yet more subtle possibilities of your chi rising and falling

6. You next will become progressively aware of more and more subtle layers and possibilities inherent within each of the 16 parts of the Taoist nei gung system that are part and parcel of the entire meaning of "sink your chi to the lower tantien."

Chi Flow and Tai Chi Movements

Each individual posture (movement) has specific chi flows associated with it, as do four or more linked moves. The chi flows of these linked movements have specific internal rhythms, which altogether create a certain kind of chi. Small series of movements simultaneously benefit the body's overall chi in specific ways, just as individual postures create specific chi flows within particular parts of the body.

Intermittently you may get spontaneous insights into how specific flows work. Initially, however, impressions are usually more vague and imprecise, or just out of reach. You sense you know but aren't quite sure how.

You can make your chi flow in various specific ways. For example:

- inside to outside, outside to inside
- up to down, down to up
- left to right, right to left
- towards or away from the spine, lower tantien, or central channel of energy
- within the energetic space or aura around your body
- between the physical body and the boundary of the aura.

These energy flows in you can externally affect observers. Animals often stop and watch transfixed or come close to suck up the energy. It usually helps people who are sick feel better and often speeds up their healing process when someone practices in their room. Chi flows may stay focused only within the physical body to the edges your skin, or may extend into the external space around your body, commonly called the bioelectric field, etheric body, or aura.

The 16-Part Nei Gung System

The Taoist science of how these energy flows work is called the 16-part nei gung system. These energy techniques were discovered and developed by Taoist monks as they delved deeply into their minds and bodies during meditation. They developed chi-energy to maintain superior health, heal illness, and realize profound inner stillness and spirituality. Later their work created nei gung, which became what is often called chi gung today and formed the energetic foundation of the internal martial arts of tai chi, hsing-i, and ba gua.

These ancient methods, which have been kept relatively secret for millennia, have immense depths. With good teachers, they may be communicated on a surface, medium, or very deep level. Each one of the components of nei gung could legitimately merit a very large book of its own. Each component forms a segment of a continuous circle, where there is no definitive starting or ending point, and each is organically connected to the rest. The order is not fixed and linear, only descriptive. As it is impossible to state the precise beginning or end of a circle, so the 16 components also have neither a beginning nor end point. As such, each and every time you go around the circle of 16, it becomes possible to go to a deeper, more fulfilling, and beneficial level with each individual component.

The complete nei gung system can be made accessible for an ordinary person, although it is generally only known or taught by masters of tai chi martial arts, Taoist chi gung, or meditation. Any individual tai chi school may know or teach none of the components, a few of them, or all of them. Some are comfortable teaching the 16-part nei gung system openly, others only in secret.

The 16 parts are:

1. Breathing methods, from the simple to the complex. In regular breathing, your belly expands as you inhale and shrinks when you exhale. In reverse breathing, you do the opposite—shrink your belly when you inhale and expand it when you exhale. *Every* anatomical part and energetic function within your body and external aura will get larger and smaller in coordination with the expansions and contractions of your belly

2. Causing chi to travel along all the various ascending, descending, and lateral connecting channels within the body. The whole process includes methods to help you feel your chi so that you can move it smoothly to where it will work most efficiently for varying purposes. Part of this is concerned with how to transform or dissolve and release the qualities of the energies flowing within specified channels

3. Precise body alignments to prevent the flow of chi from being either blocked or dissipated. From a Western perspective, practicing these principles brings about exceptionally effective biomechanical alignments

The Energy Anatomy of the Body

reprinted from *The Power of Internal Martial Arts*

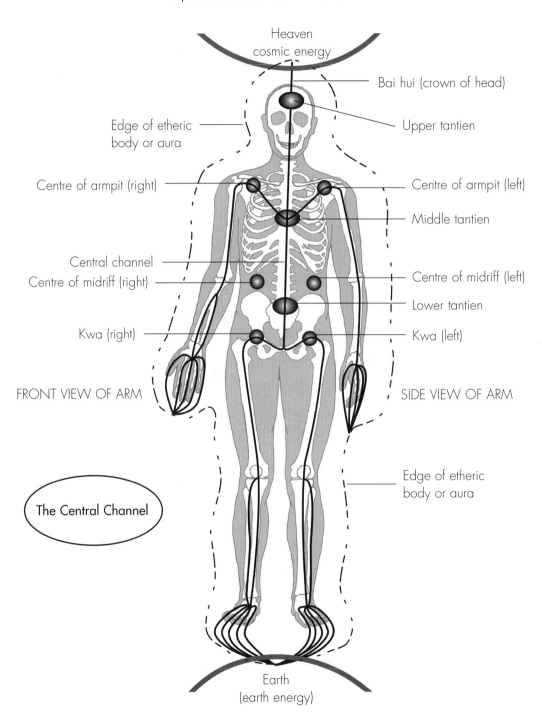

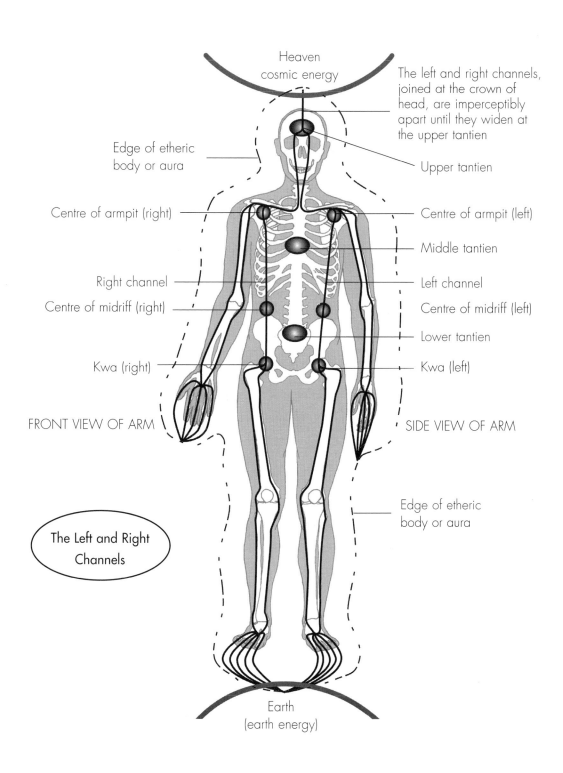

Heaven cosmic energy

The left and right channels, joined at the crown of head, are imperceptibly apart until they widen at the upper tantien

Edge of etheric body or aura

Upper tantien

Centre of armpit (right)

Centre of armpit (left)

Middle tantien

Right channel

Left channel

Centre of midriff (right)

Centre of midriff (left)

Lower tantien

Kwa (right)

Kwa (left)

FRONT VIEW OF ARM

SIDE VIEW OF ARM

Edge of etheric body or aura

The Left and Right Channels

Earth (earth energy)

4. Dissolving, releasing, and resolving all blockages of the physical, emotional, and spiritual sides of yourself

5. Moving chi-energy through the main and secondary acupuncture channels, energy gates and points, as well as a multitude of tiny channels that cause specific functions to occur. Many of these are not widely known in the West[4]

6. Bending and stretching the body's soft tissues from the inside out, and from the outside in, and along the direction of the body's yin and yang acupuncture channels

7. Opening and closing methods. Opening means to expand, grow larger, or flow outwards and emanate like a sun. Closing means to condense inwards, and get smaller along an inward direction of motion, like the gravity flow of a black hole or dwarf star. Closing carries no connotation of tension, contraction, or force in the movement, only continuous inward flow toward a point of origination, like iron filings moving toward a magnet. Opening and closing actions can occur within any of the body's soft and hard physical tissues. Equally, opening and closing can occur anywhere within the body's subtle energy anatomy (channels, points, aura, etc.)

8. Working with the energies of the external aura, as they interchange and connect both with the contents of the physical body and non-physical mental states; equally, going beyond the personal to the connections between the physical body, aura, and the rest of the psychic and spiritual forces and flows that exist within the universe

9. Generating circles and spirals of energy inside your body that have been almost entirely dormant, as well as amplifying and controlling the flow of these currents that are already naturally operating well

10. Moving chi to any part of your body at will (especially the internal organs, glands, and spots within the brain and spinal cord). This includes absorbing or projecting chi from any body part at will

11. Awakening and controlling all the energies of the spine, and what they connect to. This includes the vertebrae, cerebrospinal fluid, and the spinal cord itself

12. Awakening and using the body's left and right energy channels

13. Awakening and using the body's central energy channel, which ultimately controls all the others

14. Developing the capacities and all the uses of the body's lower tantien, the main

---

[4] The entire, immensely complex Taoist science of chi works with thousands of specific channels, each with specific and interconnected functions.

energetic center that directly affects all physical functions, our sense of bodily fear or insecurity, including death, and our sense of being stable and grounded in this world

15. Developing the capacities and all the uses of the body's middle and upper tantien, the "higher" human spiritual centers. The middle tantien, also called the heart center, governs all relationships. It is intimately tied to all our most subtle emotions and intuitions, and is considered the source of consciousness within the body. The upper tantien, located within the brain, is critical to longevity because of its ability to activate the master glands of the body, the pituitary and pineal glands. It is also responsible for well-functioning thought processes and potential psychic capacities

16. Integrating and connecting each of the previous 15 components into one unified energy, physically and otherwise. Permanent integration is different from a temporary buzz, or having a lot of energy that generates strong experiences but ultimately goes nowhere. Lacking number 16, it is difficult to absorb and integrate the good qualities of the other 15 in a stable and comfortable manner that allows you to use them effortlessly to maximum effect—such as when you are not thinking about them, while resting, or during sleep.

It is useful to recognize that being able to create a temporary energetic state is different from stabilizing it within you, so in extreme need you can call on it easily at will. Integration allows the nei gung within tai chi to give you its maximum potential smoothly and easily throughout daily life.

Opening and Closing

To quote Men Hui Feng, the former head of tai chi instructors at the Beijing Center of China's state tai chi certification system, "Without opening and closing, there is no tai chi."

For the average person the opening and closing methods for internally and externally expanding and contracting are very counterintuitive, especially because neither muscular nor any other kind of tension is to be employed. These openings and closings are achieved through relaxation and having the movements flow either towards or away from a point of origination.

Embodying these levels of physical, mental, and energetic relaxation is a challenge that everyone must undergo to progress through each stage of tai chi's more advanced levels. Opening and closing techniques are essential to understanding the implications of yin and yang in tai chi.

As your arms extend and retract during all tai chi movements, the most obvious visible, external example of opening and closing occurs within the changing size of the soft crook of your elbow, as it rhythmically alternates between becoming larger (opening) and smaller (closing). Internally, the usual invisible starting point of opening and closing occurs when you use your intent to influence the motions of the synovial fluid inside your joints to open and close them.

The synovial fluid lubricates the joints and, as they move within their natural range of motion, helps ensure that there is a buffer between the bones. You can test this range of motion by holding one end of the joint stable, and then pulling (opening) or pushing (closing) the other end. If you do not exceed 100 percent of the joint's range, you should normally experience no pain or discomfort. Exceeding this natural boundary, however, can cause problems to arise. While practicing tai chi you should never lock

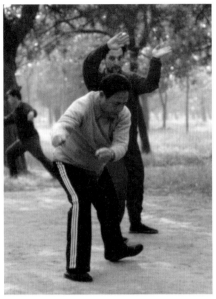

Caroline Frantzis

In tai chi, opening and closing techniques continuously alternate and flow into each other. Opening and closing is externally the most obvious in the Chen style, and less noticeable or even invisible in other styles. Here the author does the opening part of a movement sequence while Chen Style Master, Feng Zhi Qiang, does the closing phase

your joints or put them in an extremely open or closed position (beyond 100 percent). Joints in such a position are easily dislocated or broken during self-defense situations, or while stiffening up your body during a car crash.

These extremes not only violate the 70 percent rule but, even more importantly, render you incapable of using and reaping the benefits of tai chi's opening and closing techniques. As you do tai chi, the final 30 percent of space within a joint must remain open and free, fully filled with fluid, at the end point of either an opening or a closing, in accordance with the 70 percent rule.

When first learning to open and close the joints, the common tendency of a practitioner is to make clear linear distinctions: "Now I am clearly opening the joint; now I am clearly closing the joint." In time, however, the openings and closings become more circular as the ends and beginnings of all opening/closings seamlessly flow into each other.

When done properly, opening and closing the joints of the body enables you to pressurize the movements of the synovial fluid, which results in a gentle and regular pulsing of the joints and noticeable sensations. As these pulsations become more powerfully felt, they can create a warm pleasant wave, which can spread from the joint to the entire body. In time, the deliberate pulsing of the joints will extend beyond your practice and result in this pulsing automatically and naturally continuing in a healthy, rhythmic fashion throughout the day.

Pulsing the joints has a number of benefits:

- Anatomically, pulsing creates greater fluid movement within the joint. This both relieves pain and discomfort and makes the joint stronger and more flexible. Energetically, pulsing activates the specific energy gate within your body's energetic anatomy that helps regulate the joint's normal healthy functioning
- Pulsing in one joint can cause the next joint connected to it to pulse in sympathetic rhythm. This can happen either in a line, for example pulsing the fingers or toes can create a wave that can sequentially influence internal movement within the joints to the end of the arms (shoulder joints), or legs (hip sockets). Alternatively, the sympathetic pulsation wave can move in two directions at once; for example, from the elbow to the shoulder and hand, or from the knee to the hip and foot. Eventually this allows all the body's joints to move in unison, fulfilling a central principle of the *Tai Chi Classics*, "One part moves, all parts move; one part stops, all parts stop"
- Increased presence of these pulsations can help heal injured joints faster and prevent or reverse arthritis or rheumatism. Conversely, lack of these pulsations can inhibit healing or cause natural body functions to degenerate
- For achieving high performance in the martial arts, closing actions are energetically essential to all its yielding or defensive techniques, and opening methods help increase its attacking or *fa jin* (see p. 236) qualities.

Once you learn how to use opening and closing techniques with your joints, you will be taught how to use them to affect physical and energetic movements to improve the functioning of virtually all your other body systems, such as:

- breath
- muscles
- ligaments and tendons
- blood vessels
- blood, lymphatic, and interstitial fluids
- fluids within and around the spine and brain
- internal organs
- glands.

Eventually you will be taught to incorporate pulsing methods into many components of the 16-part nei gung system, or other techniques within Taoist tai chi. These include continuously pulsing between:

- a specific tantien and the body's extremities
- the physical body and the boundary of the etheric body (aura)
- the boundary of the etheric body to the universe
- any yin-yang relationship within the body
- empty and full, or emptiness and form, in either martial or Taoist tai chi.

Separate and Combine

Westerners live in a fundamentally linear society, where progress is measured by achieving quantifiable goals. It is easy to adopt this mentality when learning tai chi, which is initially taught as a series of step-by-step, relatively separate linear techniques.

But for practitioners to advance, tai chi's linear techniques must be combined and integrated until they become circular and/or spherical and emanate from one undifferentiated, internal center. If this is so, the internal and external movements will be relaxed and smooth, without stops or starts. It is not that a hand makes a circle in the air in coordination with the movement of the foot, but that the hand is no longer differentiated from any part of the body, the mind, or the spirit, but is simply encompassed within your undifferentiated internal center. Everything is seamlessly integrated within that one movement in terms of its effect on body, mind, and spirit—for example, your intent both moves the hand and coordinates the hand movement with the energy flows that are generated within the body and the external aura.

When you discover the circular and spherical nature of tai chi within yourself, you will begin to understand what is meant by the 16th component of the nei gung system: integration. Although the outside of a circle or sphere is smooth and has no differentiated edges, points, or planes, it seamlessly encompasses all linear points, with no starting, stopping, or separation. This allows you to have a sense of moving only from within an internal center. The sense of individual techniques and of linear progression disappears.

Unfortunately, too many times, practitioners gain a false sense of accomplishment when they gain a specific technique. They get stuck in a goal-orientated mindset that does not enable them to pass beyond linear dimensions. The process by which growth occurs in any living organism is not merely a series of measurable linear progressions, but is more like the growth of an embryo from a single undifferentiated cell. As you learn tai chi at its most profound, undifferentiated core, you discover that you can strongly influence, realize, and increase your potential at very profound physical, energetic, emotional, and spiritual levels.

However, before this integration can occur, specific training techniques help you to learn specific facets of the various components of the nei gung system. You may learn 40 techniques or more for any one component. For example, at the beginning of your learning curve, you will learn to use the various techniques of breathing to accomplish specific, quantifiable, linear goals. For example, they could include how to specifically move the insides of your body, both in coordination with each inhale and exhale and with any external or internal physical movement you may make. Ideally within all movements, all the separate breathing techniques relate to and build upon each other, either tangentially or directly. However, at the end of the learning curve, after learning all the layering that encompasses the multiple aspects of breathing, all that remains is one component, number 1, of the nei gung system—breathing.

When separate breathing techniques cease to be the mind's focus, then breathing, physical movement, and energy become undifferentiated. They are seamlessly integrated into all aspects of the tai chi form from the very center of your internal being and awareness. If anything untoward happens during some specific linear movement, that center point of your being instantaneously recognizes, adjusts, and corrects it, without needing to break the internal flow.

The process of separate and combine is repeated for each of the first 15 nei gung components individually. In time, any two components combine to become one integrated, circular or spherical whole controlled by your internal center point. You then combine three components, then four, etc., until all 15 become a circular whole. Each increase in the number combined brings a quantum leap in your practice. Each new whole truly exceeds the sum of its parts.

This linear-circular-spherical process repeats within all the layers of the three treasures—body, energy, and spirit—until they are seamlessly integrated from your internal center. The specific phrase in the *Tai Chi Classics* that defines this process is called "first separate then combine." The "combine" part is the 16th and final truly spherical component of the nei gung system.

This is the magic of tai chi. Without the absolute sense of what it is to take the separate linear techniques you have learned and combine and integrate them within yourself circularly or spherically, you cannot become an advanced tai chi practitioner.

Fa Jin—Projecting Power

Fa Jin is an essential part of all internal martial arts practices. Fa jin means to discharge, release, throw out, or project power. Depending on the development level of the practitioner, fa jin exists in a continuum between physical and chi-energy practices.

The openings, closings, and twistings of the body create internal compressions and releases, which in turn develops fa jin, the discharging of energy.

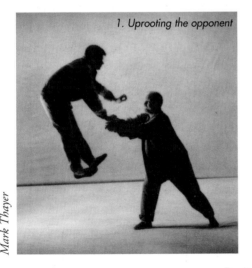
1. Uprooting the opponent

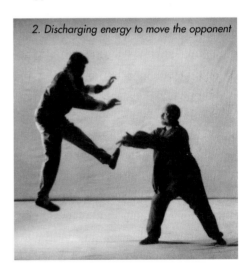
2. Discharging energy to move the opponent

Mark Thayer

Fa Jin Techniques

Whereas most martial arts use physical strength and muscular force to achieve their power, tai chi and other internal martial arts do not. Power is achieved in total relaxation, without muscular tension, by using fa jin techniques. These techniques release energy (chi) in short concentrated bursts that create tremendous power. This power can pass through an attacker's body, bringing him no physical damage or pain, but causing his body to be thrown several feet away as if picked up by a gust of wind. Alternatively, the force of fa jin can be concentrated inside the attacker's body, where the energy released can cause serious harm.

The critical issue in fa jin is the storage and sudden release of energy at a specific point in time and space. This technique may be introduced to beginning students, but is more appropriately explored by intermediate and advanced students during push hands and martial art training. If fa jin is done *gently* during the tai chi form (rather than during push hands or in fighting), it benefits your health by releasing the body's stagnant chi. (See Chapter 3, p. 59.)

The *Tai Chi Classics*

Learning to fully understand and implement the principles embedded in the *Tai Chi Classics* is central to succeeding in tai chi's intermediate and advanced aspects (see Chapter 9 for its historical origins). Without incorporating these principles within your own practice, the full potential of tai chi cannot emerge. They are the meat of both tai chi's external and internal movements.

The *Tai Chi Classics* contain series of short, terse, sometimes opaque, poetic, phrases, for example, "from posture to posture the internal energy is unbroken." Each phrase is composed of four Chinese characters, which do not translate well into literal English or other Western languages.

Because of the emphasis on finding a good teacher in the *Tai Chi Classics*, most teachers in China start introducing phrases appropriate to the level of a beginner's understanding fairly early on. This is because all the phrases are, by nature, very multi-level, so much so that they are equally relevant for the novice and the most proficient master.

Although many authors elaborate on the meanings of the phrases, none of them really go into the full range of what they mean. Their progressively deeper meanings often cannot be fully understood through common sense or intellectual extrapolation but must be experienced within the tai chi movements. The deeper meanings of each phrase require specific new knowledge to interpret, implement and, understand. Until a person diligently practices, ponders, and draws the meaning out of his or her own depths, the meaning will remain secret, regardless of how clearly it is verbally explained.

The meanings of each phrase will unfold and deepen as a person practices. If you want to become an advanced student, you must find out (1) what the primary and tangential meanings of each phrase are; (2) learn about the specific training methods that implement each phrase; and (3) learn how each of the different phrases are subtly interlinked and build upon each other.

Each phrase could be used to cover only one specific principle in a specific context. More commonly, however, each phrase is interconnected and directly linked to many other phrases within the classics in webs of intricate, integrated, and useful information. The complete story about some very large topic could be embedded in ten or more phrases dispersed throughout the *Tai Chi Classics*. These topics might be:

- chi cultivation directly applicable to health, healing, and longevity
- Taoist philosophy, psychology, and spirituality
- strategies for handling conflict in general, which are directly applicable for higher-level martial arts or the world of business, sports, or government.

Each individual phrase could have very different implications depending upon whether you are looking at them from the viewpoint of body, energy, or spirit.

Some examples of the ideas in the *Tai Chi Classics* could include:

Physical principles:
- shoulders stay down rather than raised
- spine is straight not slumped or arched
- waist moves the hands rather than vice versa
- waist and legs are fully connected and move as one unit
- the body should be without bulges or hollows
- one part moves, all parts move; one part stops, all parts stop.

Energetic principles:
- mind leads and the chi follows
- chi moves through the body like the thread between a string of nine pearls
- chi descends from your spine, to your waist, legs, and feet, through and below the ground
- chi begins in the feet, and moves through the legs and waist, spine and arms, and expresses itself through the finger tips
- chi sticks to the spine

- empty and full must be clearly differentiated
- storing energy is like bending a bow, releasing energy is like shooting an arrow
- the neck is empty and the internal chi rises to above the head, and holds the head suspended.

Spiritual principles:
- from posture to posture the internal power is unbroken
- the spirit should be collected within
- yang does not leave yin, yin does not leave yang.

Martial and strategic principles:
- seize the moment and take the opportunity
- one's mind during the form should be like a hawk waiting to seize a rabbit
- four ounces deflects a thousand pounds
- I begin after my opponent, but arrive before him.

Many tai chi books in European and Asian languages contain sections on the *Tai Chi Classics*. Different authors have either more basic or profound insights into the ways they interpret the various phrases within it. Some books mention some essential phrases, but not others. Within China most of the more respected authors would not seriously consider tackling the *Classics* until they had extensively practiced tai chi and chewed on its deeper meanings for at least thirty years.

How to Practice for High-Level Performance

To go beyond simply being free from illness to developing superior physical, mental, and spiritual functioning, tai chi becomes increasingly more complex and challenging. Usually the progression goes from easier health practices, to general overall fitness, to martial arts, to pushing the envelope to encompass maximum physical speed, power, vitality, mental clarity, and spiritual potential. Besides the form, you learn other techniques such as push hands, sparring barehanded and with weapons (mainly swords, spears, and poles), and basic meditation techniques either incorporated within the form, or others done standing and sitting. If your interest is to achieve spiritual potential, extensive seated meditation at ever more profound levels would be alternated with the moving tai chi form. In a few traditions, the full range of techniques for tai chi as a martial art would also be added to the spiritual mix.[5]

To obtain optimum performance you will need to learn and embody the 16-part nei gung system in greater depth for two basic reasons. First, to maximize the amount of exercise, chi flow, and power each minute of your practice time will generate. Second, to prevent unnecessary injuries, which reduce your ability to train and use up valuable time in recovery. Or, at the most extreme level, injuries could compromise your abilities for life, as often happens to competitive athletes who get so damaged that they must retire entirely and suffer lifelong pain.

High performance will eventually require doing the tai chi form both in extremely slow motion and with lightning fast speed. It will demand many things, including agility, flexibility, physical power training using subtle chi methods, and the ability to stand on one leg for extended periods.

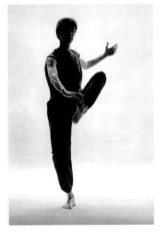

If you wish to add self-defense techniques to the mix, applications done at slow and medium speed are sufficient for health, while full-speed rapidly changing defense maneuvers are necessary for full fitness. To perform tai chi in a superior manner under the pressures of combat, or adapt it to the extreme rigors of competitive sports or business requires very consistent training. It demands that you upgrade your internal organs, glands, and joints in order to deliver superior vitality and mental alertness. All of this has to be combined with a mind and central nervous system that are relaxed, calm, flexible, and able to recover from stress rapidly.

Repulse Monkey from the Wu style long form. This movement is difficult in terms of physical balance. It is integral to many of the throwing techniques of the Wu style

How Much, Where, and When to Practice

For high performance you need to practice at least one to two hours daily.

However, the issue of high performance begs the question of how healthy or fit you wish to be. It should be mentioned that a quality of fitness that makes your body and mind ever more strong yet relaxed is quite different than fitness that makes your body and mind ever more tense, albeit strong.

If you have a busy working life, doing the form an hour daily most days a week will usually give you the maximum high performance benefits without violating the 70 percent rule and

---

[5] See *The Power of Internal Martial Arts* (North Atlantic Books, 1998), Chapter 1, which covers the animal, human, and spiritual approaches to martial arts.

creating excess stress and strain. For most people under sixty with a lot of free time, two hours of solo form work daily is about the maximum amount of recommended practice time. Partner practices such as push hands could then be added on top, according to your interest and scheduling considerations.

For those who wish to attain the highest level of achievement, the issue becomes what is the maximum, productive time you can spend, without over-training and exceeding the 70 percent rule and thereby expending unproductive effort. Over-training in tai chi, like in all sports, can lead to burnout and the tendency toward injury due to exhaustion, which unravels the benefits of practice.

As a general guideline in terms of solo form work, barehanded or with traditional weapons, the absolute maximum practice time for a fit person so "you can be all you can be" reaches a point of diminishing returns. Nowadays this is usually:

- before the age of thirty—six hours daily
- between thirty and fifty—four hours a day
- between fifty and seventy—two hours a day
- after age seventy—less than two hours a day, with one hour being the most common.

The best time to practice is between two to two-and-a-half hours before sunrise. The next best time is at sunrise, to gather yang chi, and sunset to gather yin chi. However, as these times may be impractical for many, you should practice when and wherever possible. If you are appropriately attired, hot or cold environments need not be a problem. It is good to practice in the cleanest air available.

Stay out of strong winds or wear clothing that blocks it. Cold, damp places are best avoided. Also it is not recommended to practice tai chi around physically or mentally ill people, unless you are highly skilled and can energetically protect yourself. Otherwise they can excessively drain your chi, or you can pattern their unhealthy, unbalanced chi within your own body without knowing it.

High Performance Teachers

To become an accomplished practitioner and gain some of tai chi's more extraordinary chi-energy benefits, you must find an expert teacher/master in these practices, who can help you learn and integrate the Taoist 16-part nei gung program within your form.

To achieve their high level of practice and teaching, before the 1940's, the best tai chi adepts engaged in the same degree of arduous physical training that today's professional athletes, dancers, and musicians do to become and stay successful. Traditionally, training four to eight hours a day for decades was quite common among famous masters. This training time is necessary to access the full range of extraordinary chi-energy possibilities inherent in tai chi chuan.

The vast majority of those who are expert in teaching tai chi for high performance come from the tai chi *chuan* or martial arts tradition. These teachers fall into two camps. The first teach with a very fierce and intense martial flavor. Fierce martial arts practices in general, and tai chi specifically, normally take you through things you might rather avoid. These include coping with extreme aggression, both within yourself and others, exposure to physical injury, and confronting your deepest and often hidden emotions and psychological fears.

Other teachers are willing and able to teach tai chi's high performance aspects, but do so with a lighter martial arts flavor. This allows them to keep it real in terms of tai chi's health and high performance enhancement capacities, but without undue emphasis on fighting and combative practices.

Conclusion

Tai chi is a lifetime learning experience. Be patient with yourself. Patience is a virtue that tai chi brings out in people, something much needed in this age of anxiety.

Remember that the greed for knowledge can easily make you obsessed and do silly things, as well as cause you to violate the 70 percent rule. However, the more you put into tai chi, the more its gifts will continually unfold and benefit your life.

To quote my late mentor Liu Hung Chieh, "Whatever you practice over time, you become."

12 Choosing a Teacher

My hope in this chapter is to clarify what a master really is—at a very high level—as the term is used in China.

If Western teachers know what is possible, over time, teachers will try to establish equally high standards in the West. If students know what they are looking for, they can know what to ask for, saving them from going down false roads or not achieving their full potential.

Someone with little experience of tai chi might watch a tall, attractive person doing tai chi and exclaim, "What a graceful dance." However, to many serious teachers or long-term practitioners, such a statement would be an insult—implying that their practice was fluff and not coming from the core within their body and mind.

It would also be insulting to say, "Tai chi looks so hypnotic." This would mean that the teacher or practitioner was not awake and aware. One of tai chi's goals is to produce a person who is simultaneously relaxed and totally aware, whether exercising, fighting, engaged in business negotiations, competitive sports, or whatever.

This is the dilemma that confounds many inexperienced people looking for a tai chi teacher. They do not understand that tai chi is

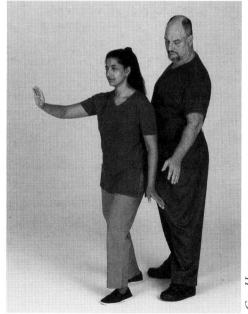

Guy Hearn

Correcting a student's posture first requires careful observation. Then the instructor makes gentle and precise adjustments. The posture shown here, Brush Knee, Twist Step, *is common to almost all tai chi forms*

a very sophisticated and carefully constructed body-mind training, which with practice deepens and has a profound effect on health, emotions, and longevity. It affects the insides of the body and mind in ways that are not obvious and even counterintuitive to those who have not learned it from a good teacher.

More is required of a skilled tai chi teacher than one teaching an intellectual skill, such as mathematics or English. When students are working with chi development and personal internal growth, intellectual knowledge alone is insufficient. The level of the teachers' personal accomplishments also determines their capacity to transmit these qualities to another. The universal spiritual qualities of teaching intricate body-mind relationships mandate that teachers be able to embody and communicate the qualities they teach non-verbally. If their chi is not full and relaxed, then it is unlikely that their students' chi will become so.

To obtain tai chi's valuable and long-lasting benefits, choosing a skilled teacher is key. This is ultimately more important in learning any aspect of tai chi than the specific style the teacher does. Unfortunately, there is no equivalent to a consumer's guide to help you choose among the thousands of tai chi instructors and the few masters currently teaching in the West. Levels of competence vary greatly and your choices will likely contain many trade-offs.

There are no simple criteria for determining competence. To make this issue more complicated, the criteria for determining a teacher's competence for a beginner is very different than those for an advanced student.

The four basic issues that generally define "better" are: 1) the quality of the teacher's knowledge (competence); 2) the teacher's ability to communicate, both verbally and non-verbally; 3) their decency, honesty, and generosity; and 4) the student's comfort level with the teacher. Most students who choose and stay with a tai chi teacher will define why they like that teacher in one or more of these terms. If you have teachers with the same innate talent, the ones that are decent, honest, and generous are likely to take you further and upgrade your knowledge faster, since tai chi is an activity that deals so directly with the human spirit.

However, if you must choose between an ordinary teacher you are comfortable with and an excellent but somewhat less personable teacher, in my opinion, choose excellence. In general, the quality of instruction will be remembered long after the price of learning is forgotten, or as the old maxim goes, "you get what you pay for."

A competent tai chi teacher can positively influence you and possibly change your life for the better. Incompetent ones can turn you off forever.

Benchmarks for Beginners

Although everyone would love to begin studying with a master, for a variety of positive and negative reasons, most beginners do not need to do so. You do not initially need to learn piano from a world-class concert pianist to enjoy the benefits of playing the piano or to understand whether you want, or have the talent, to become such a world-class pianist. Particularly for beginners, the basics that are outlined in Chapter 10 can be effectively taught by many tai chi teachers, whether ordinary or quite exceptional. By practicing regularly you will begin to acquire the health and relaxation benefits of tai chi.

However, the better the teacher, the faster the students who are exceptionally committed will learn and absorb what is being taught, and the more motivated they will be to continue their practice. If this is you, take the time to seek out exceptional teachers that are right for you and can help you advance more quickly.

If you have yet to take a tai chi class, read this book carefully so that you understand the benefits tai chi can provide. Remember that this lifelong practice requires effort to learn and looks easier than it is. Here are some guidelines that will help you choose the teacher who is right for you:

- Consider what goals you want to achieve
- Apply some simple competence gauges
- Evaluate the instructors' teaching experience and their ability to communicate
- Understand the differences between styles/frames/forms and how they may apply to you
- Think about which teaching approach works best for you and which personality types you can work with.

You should also visit some tai chi classes and talk with students about some of the issues covered in this chapter. The goal is to find a teacher who works for you and helps you gain the benefits for which tai chi is justifiably renowned.

Credentials

Contrary to popular myth, tai chi does not have black belts or other obvious visible signs of competence. Nevertheless in China, there is a long-established hierarchy of learning and teaching (see p. 259—China's Five Levels of Competence—later in this chapter).

Western countries have no equivalent to the Chinese system for testing competence. There are no generally recognized rating and accreditation systems, no consumer guides, no uniforms or belts. Although some masters are beginning to issue teaching credentials to students who have passed instructor trainings, the vast majority of available tai chi teachers lack such credentials.

In the West, many teachers will allude to their competence by stating how long they have done tai chi and referencing their teachers. Although some may have studied with high level people and practiced for many years, they may still be incompetent or poor practitioners and teachers. Moreover, just because a teacher has a Chinese or Asian name does not automatically confer competence, nor does the fact that a Westerner has studied with a Chinese or Asian practitioner. There is usually no practical way for most people to check the credentials of a teacher. This can make it difficult for students who want to study with an exceptional teacher or master to find one.

Currently the tai chi, chi gung, and yoga worlds are struggling with the issues of whether teacher credentials should be issued, through what organizational mechanisms, and by what standards. In yoga, for example, they are questioning whether it is even proper to credential a "spiritual subject." In tai chi's case, the Chinese language barrier is a further complication. The issues are complex and for at least the first decade of the twenty-first century, resolution of them seems unlikely.

Consider your Goals

After reading this book, you may have determined that you want to learn tai chi for one or more reasons, which may include:

- relaxation and stress reduction
- improved health and wellness
- longevity
- joy of movement
- entertainment and socialization
- learning an unusual and challenging body/mind/spirit practice
- self-defense
- putting more chi-energy in your life
- spirituality and personal growth.

Perhaps you want to enhance your life or address specific health issues, such as high blood pressure, pain management, prevention or alleviation of carpal tunnel or other repetitive stress injuries, or recovery from an accident or operation. Perhaps you need a teacher skilled at teaching the handicapped or the elderly.

You need to tell potential teachers what you specifically want to achieve and ask if they can help you rather than assuming that they can. Not all teachers may be able or willing to teach what you need or desire to learn.

The more specific your requirements, the more experience your teacher needs to have. For example, if you are interested in self-defense, you should study with someone who can teach you the applications for each movement and how to apply them in threatening situations. To enhance physical or intellectual performance, you need someone who thoroughly knows and is experienced in internal power and developing the 16-part nei gung system (see p. 226). If you have a specific health problem, it is best to find someone experienced in dealing with that problem or related ones.

No one can teach you what they have not learned themselves.

Therapy

Some tai chi teachers work better with sick people than others; some work better with specific types of illnesses and physical ailments. If you wish to use tai chi as self-therapy for a specific problem, it is important that the instructor's bedside manner or personality works for you and doesn't turn you off. Otherwise you may find it psychologically difficult to practice on your own, an essential component for your recovery.

The most effective teachers for self-therapy have personally used tai chi to recover from serious illness or injury. Having been through it themselves, they know the pitfalls, and how to apply the 70 percent rule. They can truly empathize and have insight into how to overcome the inevitable psychological and physical hardships the healing process engenders—walking the razor's edge between frustration and patience, pain and healing.

It is best is to find an instructor who has personally managed to heal an illness or injury with tai chi and has professional experience in adapting it for therapeutic purposes. These teachers are rare, because it is hard to get the training and clinical experience in the West. However, because this area of tai chi is getting more attention, more instructors are getting involved, and consequently, over time, an increasing supply of qualified personnel should emerge.

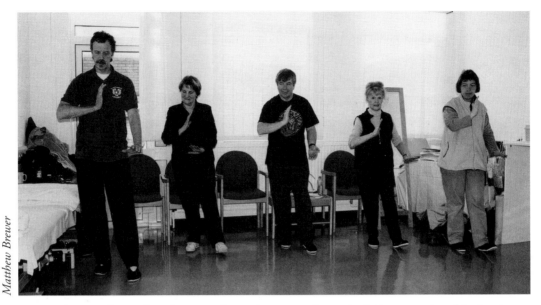

Matthew Breuer

Brian Cookman teaches tai chi at the Kent and Canterbury Hospital in England. He is a member of the Steering Group for the UK Tai Chi and Chi Gung Forum for Health and Special Needs. "I have been working for four years at the first UK hospital to use tai chi as a complementary therapy. I teach people who are suffering from multiple sclerosis, chronic fatigue, rheumatism, arthritis, heart conditions, unresolved pain—basically anyone the doctors cannot further help. They give me their notes and details and I try to work out what is best for them. Their improvement is dramatic and many have reduced their medications. Amazing."

Gauging Competence

Tai chi can only be learned from someone who is a competent practitioner. In order for you to obtain tai chi's extraordinary benefits, your teachers themselves must possess them, including such intangible qualities as mental and emotional clarity and relaxation.

Generally, if you are a beginner, many practitioners will have the competence to teach basic body mechanics and alignments, how to execute the moves with relaxation and make sure you understand elementary safety techniques. Until the basics have been mastered, you will lack the necessary foundation to successfully absorb the more advanced techniques, such as going deeply inside the body, developing circularity of movement and developing chi.

Earlier chapters have covered a great deal of information about what tai chi can offer and what you can expect to learn during various stages. Some teachers are able to teach these stages; some can only talk about them. Here is a hierarchy of some of the less technical ways you can gauge competence, even if you have never taken a tai chi class.

1. The teachers must be present, aware, and relaxed when doing the form
2. Their movements must be smooth, continuous, and fluid
3. They must *never* lock or straighten any of their joints
4. Their body must move as a connected, aligned, and integrated whole, without some body parts seeming to move independently
5. The teachers must have a lot of relaxed chi-energy.

Experience Counts

The three kinds of experience that are important are time spent studying, time spent doing, and time spent teaching. It takes time and experience to understand how to teach almost anything effectively. How much and what experience does the teacher have?

This is a difficult area to address because actual time spent studying, doing, or teaching does not always equate with competence. That someone *should be* good and that they *are* good don't always fit. Studying something doesn't say if you learned it well or even at all.

Even for the very talented, from the original point of learning with a master it can take approximately ten years to "understand and fully put what you learned into your blood and bones" and gain the mature ability to fully impart the basics to a student.

Teachers usually improve if they have more study time behind them, either at the beginning or by continuously upgrading over time. This is because, like you, they are students who need to train their bodies to stretch, relax, and develop extraordinary coordination and chi.

In the West there are many who learned from a teacher for only a few months and then practiced for twenty years by themselves. Chinese masters would call these people self-taught. Generally speaking, only a few of these individuals are extremely competent practitioners, as most do not overcome the limiting conditions of an incomplete education. This does not even bring up the question of whether their original teacher was competent. Self-taught teachers may not know enough to teach you the basics correctly. So when you find a more competent teacher, you could easily spend a long time shedding bad habits.

Other teachers might say that they have cumulatively spent years, even the full two decades on a very regular basis with one or more teachers. Even if very untalented, they usually don't confuse what the basics should be.

Teaching experience is even harder to quantify. Although the same ten-year marker applies for almost all, some people never become good instructors no matter how long or how many they teach, despite the fact that they might be very competent in their own practice. Great practitioners can be wonderful, average or very poor teachers.

Most teachers improve with experience. For example, after decades of teaching, a teacher can recognize what a student needs in under a minute, whereas it may have taken them an hour or longer to correctly determine the same information in the early years. Time can also sometimes upgrade those who begin with mediocre natural teaching abilities into exceptional mentors.

There is a fairly well known example of someone in China who began as a mediocre student but eventually became an exceptional Wu style practitioner and teacher. Ma Yueh Liang (1901–1998) of Shanghai was considered in the 1920s and 1930s to be only so-so by his classmates, although married to the daughter of the founder of the Wu style. Over time, however, he became known as one of the best practitioners. Even Ma himself said that although exposed to Wu's inner teachings, it was only after over thirty years' practice that he began to uncover what Wu was really driving at. Like the ancient Greek fable of the tortoise and the hare, slow, but sure and committed, can win the race.

Finally, you need to know whether the teacher is a professional or amateur—that is, is he or she teaching primarily to make a living? Professionals usually offer a more consistent level of quality. Perhaps as important a question is whether or not a teacher is continuing to study tai chi.

Amateurs may be more erratic in their practice and in their teaching. The pressures of their regular job and daily life might cause them to miss classes, be distracted, or be focused elsewhere when they are supposed to be teaching.

Professionals tend to be more skilled and organized than most amateurs. Often they are significantly better. Since they need to make a living teaching tai chi, they have a greater stake in being competent and developing a consistently high quality product. The exceptions are the naturally talented who, when young, studied tai chi extensively with excellent teachers and continued to practice while becoming involved in an unrelated career. Such practitioners could still become excellent instructors if they decided to take up teaching tai chi even decades later.

Communication

Having competence in tai chi, "walking the talk," and being able to teach and effectively communicate it, "talking the walk," are two different skills. The best teachers combine both in one package. If several teachers seem equally competent as practitioners, pick the best communicator.

Ideally, teachers should be able to convey accurate, complete, and understandable instructions. This will help you avoid wasting time through misinterpreting what you thought you were

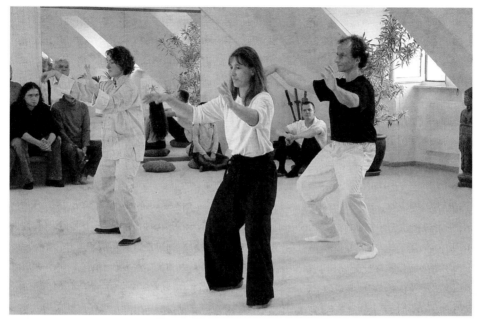

Heinz Schoppel

Instructors demonstrate Wu style tai chi at the Tai Chi Schule Neu-Ulm in Southern Germany

supposed to do. Teachers must ensure that students understand when, how, and why they may be over-extending their physical and emotional systems.

Equally important is that teachers must understand how a student learns and be able to recognize when a student is misunderstanding instructions or is misinterpreting the subtleties of what is being conveyed. Ideally, they must also realize when students are violating the 70 percent rule, are over-exciting their glands or central nervous system, are overly attracted to the rushes they might experience from the movement of chi, or ignoring the useful advice of the teacher.

Common Approaches to Teaching Tai Chi

Here are the most common ways tai chi is taught:

1. You watch and follow. The teacher does the movement. The student learns primarily by watching the teacher or senior students and mimicking the movements. Sometimes specific information on what you are supposed to do may be offered, but not often. Your imagination fills in the blanks. Many Asian

teachers start this way, some because of an inherent language barrier, and some because it was how they were taught. Although the teacher may be inspiring, technical corrections are rarely given. This approach is difficult for many beginners, particularly in the West, because they have no context for understanding why they are doing the movements and what they are supposed to avoid (such as over-extending the knee or locking the joints)

2. What you are supposed to do is broadly explained either before or after certain movements; or individual movements are broken down into their specific constituent parts (how to move the hand; when to shift the weight, what to do with your chi, etc.). Over time the instructions get deeper and more complete, enabling you to incorporate more of them into your form

3. Either in single movements or at specific points during the form, the teacher makes nonverbal corrections, perhaps by touching and molding your body and energy. Often with the most worthy students, masters will use this as a primary teaching method

4. Touch is combined with specific oral instructions

5. Some teachers communicate by inspiration and the power of their chi only. Either subtly or dramatically, they demonstrate various qualities of tai chi, but often don't overtly explain the meaning, give a coherent specific context for what they just did, or elaborate on its potential. The student must use his or her intuition to work out how it was done without help. For example, my first main internal martial arts teacher, Wang Shu Jin, depended upon his chi and personal prowess more than his explanations to teach. This approach is seldom effective for beginners. It works best only for relatively talented or more accomplished students with whom the subtle connections between teacher and student are very strong

6. Some teachers first give the big shape of movements without much explanation, and over time put flesh on the bones. However, they may or may not let you know when the pieces of the fleshing out process will be taught. Their teaching method appears random, so that you don't know what will come next. If you are absent one day, important pieces may not be repeated for years. Again, this approach works best for advanced students and not for beginners.

Consider What Style to Learn

Initially, it is best to start off with the right style and frame size for your needs, as explained in Chapter 9. This will more effectively help you move through the challenges of learning tai chi and avoid emotional and physical problems. For example, older people with little tai chi experience may want to choose a short form style. It will be quicker and simpler to learn than a long form and will be easier on your joints. A very tall, lanky person, for instance, may want to choose a large frame style.

A tai chi teacher who has been trained in one style may not be competent in teaching or even understanding a different one.

Personality and Substance

Good teachers keep your attention, especially in hard-to-understand and challenging areas. They will have different ways of accomplishing this: encouragement, forcefulness, humor, gentleness, blunt directness, non-verbal body language, etc. Some teachers use precise words to make the point clearly understood; others say more with a simple gesture than a three-hour lecture.

Many students cannot separate what is being taught from an instructor's personal teaching style. But a great personality may be a very poor tai chi practitioner. Alternatively, a teacher may have some disagreeable personal traits and be an excellent practitioner. In terms of benefiting students, it is my opinion that in tai chi, substance is ultimately more valuable than personality or teaching approach. In deciding between a charming but incompetent teacher or a highly competent teacher with some disagreeable personality traits, choose competence.

However, if you find yourself reacting too negatively to your teacher's personality, your ability to learn may be adversely impacted. For example, you may not be able to learn from someone too critical or authoritarian or too lax; or from one whose politics and religious views you cannot abide. Only you will know how to stay within your comfort zone.

Some teachers have strong emotional boundaries, which can make them seem distant, aloof, or inaccessible. Still others may use these boundaries as a defense against any extreme or dysfunctional personalities in their classes.

Some tai chi teachers go the extra mile to share their knowledge, others dole it out sparingly, if at all. The best try to maximize the benefit of tai chi to all their students and don't play favorites. They treat all their students evenhandedly, whether they like or dislike them or find them difficult to teach. A teacher's generosity of spirit often naturally translates into inspiring students and drawing out their natural abilities, so the students can acquire the practical foundation to translate their goals into realities.

It takes as much or more patience to teach tai chi as it does to learn it. Many are not very patient. Not all teachers have the patience to deal well with people's foibles and slow learning capacities. Good teachers know how to deal competently, patiently, and compassionately with disagreeable and neurotic students or those who want all the energy in the class to move towards them or to monopolize the teacher's time.

Good teachers can accept their students at whatever level of talent they present—from the naturally gifted to the physically awkward—and the best know how to deal with the more vexing human limitations.

Choosing Teachers Who Are Healthcare Professionals

Healthcare professionals who do tai chi—from doctors to body workers—have a deeper level of understanding of health issues, and are able to see how tai chi practice complements many Western and alternative medical practices. If they become teachers, they may be able to tune into this knowledge and suggest that you investigate treatments that might help you that someone not medically oriented would miss or ignore. However, medical knowledge alone will not make their tai chi any better.

In the alternative medical field, where knowledge is often acquired in two- or three-week intensive courses, you need to find out what the depth of competence is. In terms of helping you use tai chi to become healthier or to solve specific medical problems, you need to ascertain how teachers acquired their knowledge and the degree of their healing talents.

For major problems of stress, tai chi teachers who have a clinical psychology background are helpful, as they are familiar with dealing with difficult human emotions. In the same way, older, emotionally mature teachers often give a steadying hand to younger students.

Where Do I Find a Teacher?

Increasingly, tai chi is being taught in virtually every city and town in America, and more and more throughout the West. Group classes can have as few as three or four people or over a hundred participants. Many are held on an ongoing weekly basis. They occur between one and six days a week, usually during weekday evenings, or during the day on weekends. Classes tend to last from one to three hours.

Some teachers have large schools that are located in major cities and hold ongoing classes or seminars open to all. Other teachers travel and give seminars and retreats for the general public or for designated groups in corporations, government departments, associations, or hospitals. Seminars can last from a half-day to three days; retreats generally from five days to one month. Length of time for designated groups is by mutual agreement, although corporate seminars and retreats are often relatively shorter.

Venues commonly used include:

- Recreational, exercise, and sports facilities, such as private clubs, commercial health clubs, publicly funded sports centers, and YMCAs
- Universities, colleges, and community colleges, usually through physical education or philosophy departments
- Adult educational programs, along with hundreds of other courses ranging from accounting, to real estate investment, to New Age topics. Or alternative educational settings that offer seminars to the general public
- Hospitals or clinics
- Public parks
- Gymnasiums and martial arts schools, where offering tai chi for older adult students is becoming more popular, along with stretching and yoga classes
- By-the-hour rental spaces commonly found everywhere, with churches and dance studios being very common
- Community and senior centers.

Where Classes are Advertised

Places you will most likely find classes or workshops advertised include:

- Yellow pages, usually in the martial arts category, or sometimes in other sections like yoga or health
- Health, fitness, martial arts, and tai chi magazines
- Free advertising catalogs and magazines of New Age courses, like *Common Ground* in San Francisco or *Earth Star* in Boston
- The Internet, under the headings: tai chi chuan, tai chi, and tai ji quan, or sometimes qi gong, chi kung, and chi gung. Websites are especially useful for people who want to know what is happening in nearby cities

- Flyers in health food and bookstores, laundromats, restaurants, and university bulletin boards
- Paid newspaper ads are relatively rare, but free newspaper ads are commonly used.

It is generally not the best idea to try to learn tai chi's movements *solely* from a book or videotape. You need a live instructor.

Benchmarks for More Advanced Students

If your practice has advanced beyond the beginner's level, and you now want to train to a higher standard, or study a more specialized area, for example, martial arts or spiritual training, you need to find an authentic master. In China, there is a hierarchy of learning that gives people the title of "master," which makes it easier to find them. However, as with any art, exceptional tai chi teachers (masters) are, by definition, rare, and very few exist outside China.

As an old adage goes, "If you wish to become the best, train with the best." Only genuine masters can produce masters.

It is difficult to find out who are masters in the West. Since there are no credentials or consumer guides to teachers, it is much harder to know who's who than in China. Even more unfortunate is that the term "master" is more casually bestowed in the West and often lands where it does not belong.

In the West, exceptional teachers and masters are known by reputation among advanced students and teachers. However, this area is loaded with politics and many are reluctant to "name names." In general, the closer a teacher belongs in a direct line to the original founder or lineage master of a style or school, the better are the odds that they teach a more complete, as opposed to a more watered-down, version of tai chi. Therefore, when instructors state that they learned from a specific person (especially an acknowledged master or lineage holder) it has meaning. This is why lineage charts are always predominately displayed in tai chi books or articles. It is the equivalent of a resumé stating which university or scientific institute someone has attended.

In China, studying with a genuine master is considered a privilege, rather than a right. Gaining access to masters may be difficult, particularly if they only speak Chinese. Usually, you need someone personally close to a master to vouch for you or give a letter of introduction. Once introduced, you must not only be able to demonstrate proficiency and competence (judged externally and internally), but the commitment, heart, and willingness to overcome the many challenges of studying with the master. These are qualities that will be tested and judged, in both overt and subtle ways.

A few English-speaking masters live in the West. Most will not require letters of introduction or someone close to them to vouch for you, as might be the case in China. However, even when you find them, these masters may not teach in convenient locations, or be willing to teach you.

Studying with a Master or Exceptional Teacher

Studying with tai chi masters can be very inspiring. They offer a higher level of consistent quality than ordinary instructors. They can impart information not otherwise available and help you reach your goals faster. Their high level of personal accomplishment inspires you to reach for your higher potential.

Masters have the overview to see what you could easily miss and help reconcile confusions between the essential and marginal, the real and the false. Even advanced students have difficulty recognizing what are the essential or secondary points to concentrate on and practice at specific times. A master's few well-placed and timely words can be worth months of constant lectures from an ordinary instructor.

Masters have the necessary knowledge to give the best consistent advice about what, when, and how a particular aspect of tai chi is most efficient and beneficially useful for you. These concerns about quality are some reasons why tai chi people always say, "The most important thing is to get a good teacher."

Is Advanced Knowledge Being Shared?

Masters who have specific kinds of knowledge, may or may not be willing to share it with you. What will motivate a tai chi teacher to open up to you depends very much on the teacher's personality, cultural conditioning, and style. Some have an intrinsic sense of duty and generosity towards their students. Some will simply reward a student's genuine effort; others may only reward student's merit and accomplishment. Some care about their students' morals; others don't. Generally, however, the simple principle is to give if you ultimately wish to get.

To what degree masters will or won't give out knowledge depends on several factors, such as:

- the degree of their generosity of spirit
- philosophical disposition

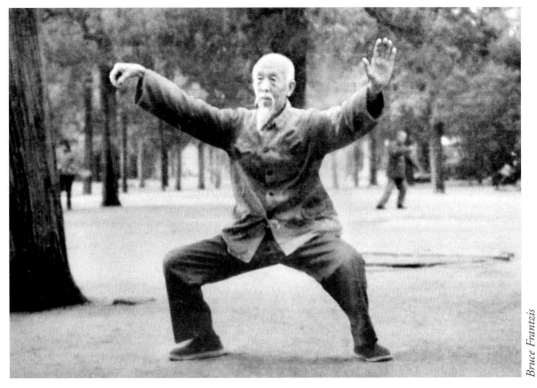

Bruce Frantzis

The author's teacher, Liu Hung Chieh, demonstrates the Single Whip posture of the Wu style

- the kind of human feeling that flows between you and them
- whether or not they play favorites based on issues besides merit
- whether or not they feel you can absorb any specific piece of knowledge at a particular moment
- whether or not they determine that your attitudes and actions show you respect tai chi and the teacher personally
- their view of your emotional, moral, or spiritual qualities.

Studying with a master, however, can be a double-edged sword. They will challenge you, sometimes without anything being said or overtly demonstrated, perhaps more than you wish to be. For some students, challenges inspire them to rise to the occasion, while for others it can be overwhelming, negatively affecting their self-esteem, and ultimately causing them to quit.

Chi-Energy Development

Although some teachers may introduce some chi-energy principles in beginning classes, chi-development occurs most strongly in intermediate and advanced classes, taught by teachers trained in the 16-part nei gung system. The better ones have been trained to teach students to progress according to their individual developmental needs.

If you want to learn chi development, you need to ask teachers if they know and are willing to teach it to you. Remember, before working with more advanced methods that can strongly develop your chi, you first need a strong foundation in tai chi's basics. Otherwise the odds are that you will ultimately fall short in your ability to develop strong chi.

China's Five Levels of Competence

In China, higher quality tai chi knowledge is acquired orally through specific teachers (individuals and their schools) and the master-disciple system, rather than state-sponsored institutions and universities. It is passed on through a well-defined hierarchical system. Students are able to define where they are in that hierarchy by the name they are given, e.g., master, disciple, senior, and junior student, etc. Being a disciple connotes a higher-level student and is the equivalent to being accepted into the top tier of Western educational institutions.

Traditionally, the most important core information was passed to only a few students, depending on their place in the hierarchy, while more peripheral information (body mechanics, movement structure, etc.) was openly and widely disseminated.

In China, students acquire five levels of knowledge during traditional tai chi education:

Level 1: Beginning students study until they are competent in the basic movements and body alignments. The overwhelming majority of China's active tai chi instructors that now teach belong to this category. Many learned tai chi through China's state-sponsored sports systems.

Level 2: Junior students study regularly for at least five years with a master, and actively practice for at least ten years. Their advancement to the next level depends on natural talent, hard work, and other factors.

Level 3: Senior students take classes with a master several days a week—if not daily—for at least a decade. Over decades some do and some do not organically develop to the level of masters.

Level 4: Masters are the *formal* disciples of lineage holders. They receive the deepest and most secretive levels of specialized knowledge available in tai chi. Masters can be truly exceptional at some but not necessarily all aspects of tai chi. Study and time practicing alone will not make a master. Unremitting effort, intense self-introspection, and a degree of natural talent are required. In China, it is said that at least thirty years are required to make a genuine master.

Masters are the superstars of tai chi, holding the equivalent of a Ph.D. and department chair at great universities. They can be compared to masters in other fields, such as basketball player Michael Jordan, dancer Mikhail Baryshnikov, and the composer Mozart.

Level 5: In a particular tai chi or school, lineage holders are disciples who over time are chosen and specifically trained in the entire tradition to hold all, not only selected parts, of the tradition and the knowledge of the previous lineage holder.

The traditional tai chi lineages had a very clear protocol regarding who was allowed to teach. Merely being a master's student did not automatically carry the master's permission to teach. In China, permission to teach could be verbally given, deliberately withheld, or not discussed by a master or by one of the senior students he or she had authorized to teach. For the quality of a teaching line to remain intact a student had to be told he could authorize others to teach, and could not take it upon him or herself to assume this was the case.

A master's permission to authorize others to teach was not casually given, either on paper or verbally with a formal ceremony. Since the master's name was behind it, it was assumed that what he knew was effectively passed to the student unless specifically cited and excluded. Classically, unless a student learned well, masters would not give them authorization to teach, as doing so diminished tai chi and insulted their own teacher's memory. Traditionally, photographs were taken with the goal to make a statement ranking the relative abilities of students. In these photos, the master was normally seated in the center and the better students were seated next to him or standing directly behind. Informal photos do not fit in this category.

Martial Arts

Many tai chi teachers include some martial arts applications as part of a more recreational and educational approach to helping you remember the movements. Some schools teach push hands, either with or without orientating it towards practical self-defense skills.

However, if you want to learn tai chi for self-defense and use it to protect yourself in a violent confrontation, you need a master who can walk the fighting talk. These teachers must be able to demonstrate applications for all movements and teach all the stages of martial arts outlined in Chapter 7. It is best if they teach safety protocols to prevent avoidable injuries. To learn practical self defense, you need a teacher who provides realistic combat situations and sparring with others. This can be physically or psychologically scary, and not necessarily user-friendly for some students.

Spirituality and Meditation

Many tai chi teachers consider tai chi as moving meditation and use it to instill relaxation and calmness (secular tai chi—see Chapter 8). Many teachers who approach tai chi from a spiritual standpoint bring in experiences from a variety of non-Taoist traditions and adapt them into their classes.

If, however, you are interested in learning tai chi as Taoist moving meditation, you will need a master extensively trained in this tradition by a master or lineage holder who is finely attuned to Taoist tai chi's spiritual traditions. Only masters can teach you all the steps that are outlined in Chapter 8. Masters that know the Taoist moving meditation tradition are rare both in China and the West.

Developing a Relationship of Trust

Teachers and students alike invest in each other. Trust and good feelings take time to build. Studying with one teacher over the long-term increases the odds that they will decide to open up completely and teach you all they have. The teacher has to know you and you need to take the time to get to know him or her. Since tai chi can involve helping to release emotional blockages and tension, trust needs to develop in both directions. It is to your advantage if teachers can become well-acquainted with your moods, so they know when best to impart new information, or encourage you to refine and stabilize previous material. The disadvantage is often that familiarity, intimacy, and trust can be misinterpreted or taken for granted.

Changing Teachers

There may come a time when you need a better teacher or master to advance to the next level. Or it may be that another teacher or master who takes a different approach can shake you up and help you upgrade previous areas of weakness or lost potential. However, finding that teacher may be difficult.

China has a well-respected tradition. When a teacher feels he has taught his student all he can, he either hands the student over to his own teacher, or a better fellow disciple, or recommends the student to another master he respects, and whom the teacher considers has qualities he personally lacks.

However, the West neither has this tradition nor many teachers with sufficient training to know when they cannot impart any more knowledge to their students, and, if they recognize this, whom to recommend.

Here are some suggestions for making changing teachers less disruptive, especially if you are training with a traditional tai chi teacher.

Jealousy and human possessiveness can always factor into human relations. Metaphorically speaking, some traditional teachers can be like jealous spouses when you train with someone else. Others are neutral and say nothing. Some only voice their reservations if they feel it could truly hinder your development. As we move farther and farther away from ancient times, some (but definitely not all) traditional teachers may be somewhat more flexible on this issue.

If you are studying with a more traditional tai chi instructor, and you want to study with someone else and think you *might* ever want to return to your original teacher, keep in mind that trust once lost is not easily regained. In order to mitigate potential bad feelings it is important to be diplomatic and try to save everyone's face. To successfully navigate these tricky cultural waters diplomatically often requires abandonment of Western ideas about hypocrisy and forthright honest relationships. As a Westerner who went through this for over a decade in China, I can state it is not always easy.

First and foremost, don't talk about either teacher by name or implication in the other's presence, or with their close senior students who might repeat what you say. If cornered and you must admit it, do so indirectly. Wounds that might heal will not if they are continuously reopened. Leave yourself what the Chinese call a back door—a way back into your old teacher's good graces. You could, for example, give an indirectly acceptable, or at least plausible reason why you need to go, with the possibility of returning in time. Equally be indirect with your next teacher so he doesn't lose face by being confronted that he "stole" you as a student, or shouldn't trust you because you have already proven your disloyalty.

If you are moving far away, ask your teacher diplomatically if he has anyone he could recommend you to study with. If, however, and only if, you see a subtle or overt wave of resistance or disapproval arise, *back off*. Then, let a little time pass and find someone else to ask if there is anyone the teacher respects in the new location or even someone who might be the best of the lesser lights. These face-saving forms with very traditional teachers can leave you a way back to studying with them again, without visible or invisible storm clouds in the background.

However, the tactics mentioned above may not apply at all to less traditional teachers, who might prefer a more direct approach and could even be insulted if you don't tell them the truth.

Are Oriental or Western Instructors Better?

Every race and culture produces good tai chi teachers. Unfortunately, those students that have innate prejudices or preferences for instructors of a particular race or religion will seldom be persuaded to learn from someone of a different race or culture. The truth, however, is that tai chi is a learned behavior, not one that is genetically passed on.

Many Westerners are more comfortable with teachers from their own culture; for the same reason, Chinese are generally more comfortable with Chinese teachers. Cross-cultural relationships are sometimes difficult to bridge, particularly if language becomes a barrier.

Many falsely think that Chinese instructors must know more and have better skills because tai chi comes from China. This can be true for those rare Chinese teachers who spent years with China's best masters and had the requisite talent to fully absorb what they were taught. However, it is not true for Chinese tai chi instructors with little training or talent who may have been the equivalent of poor or mediocre students in their own hierarchies.

Westerners can and have become masters of tai chi. Over the past several decades, increasing numbers of Westerners have studied tai chi in depth with some of the best Chinese masters. Some speak Chinese fluently, trained for years in China, have won major tournaments there, and have surpassed the skills and knowledge of the vast majority of Chinese and non-Chinese who are publicly teaching.

When evaluating teachers, the rule is look to their training and personal accomplishments, not their accent or the color of their skin.

Ability to Communicate

In terms of communications and language some people can teach so brilliantly on a non-verbal level that their students feel completely satisfied. Other students are frustrated by the non-verbal approach because although they can see something is going on, they don't understand what it is, and need clear explanations.

Language and cultural misunderstandings can obviously hinder teaching, and they happen in tai chi between Chinese and non-Chinese, both in funny and sad ways. At times both parties can think or assume they understand each other, when in fact they don't.

When I first began martial arts training in Tokyo and had not yet learned Japanese well, my teacher kept repeating the same instruction to me. I asked a fellow American who spoke Japanese well, "What did he say?" This person began to talk about spiritual masters and metaphysical mumbo jumbo, continuing on until I was sure he was going to speak about UFOs. Months later, another English speaker showed up and I asked him what the teacher's phrase meant. He replied, accurately, "Tuck your tailbone under and turn from the waist."

Studying with Oriental Teachers

You may find yourself studying with an Oriental teacher who seems culturally or philosophically very foreign to you. Western and Chinese, especially Confucian, models of what constitutes a "good" or "bad" attitude can differ significantly and dramatically.

Cross-cultural interactions can easily breed incredible misunderstandings and aggravations. Knowing and understanding that people don't think alike, nor should they, is a major challenge when trying to achieve smooth human relations across cultures.

Generally, human affection, respect for hard work and for the teacher, and a sense of the ultimate good for the group and the art of tai chi, helps bridge this divide. Almost universally, kindness, generosity, respect, deference, and caring help teachers from different cultures open up to you. And it is almost always acceptable to be neutral and diplomatic. To paraphrase Thumper's mother in the Disney cartoon, *Bambi*, "If you can't say something nice, don't say anything at all." Before most traditional masters will open up and even entertain the idea of fully sharing their innermost secrets, they must first judge if a student is honorable, moral, and loyal both to the tradition and their teacher. Whether or not continuous interpersonal contact would be retained, after a student had accepted significant training from a teacher, respect was expected for life. Loyalty was a life-long bond, where the traditional culturally-implied contract went way beyond the specific years that the transmitting of knowledge occurred.

Teacher–student perspectives can mirror Chinese perspectives concerning traditional patriarchal family relationships. Here, those above had obligations to care for, love, and nurture (teach) those below. To be considered good students, those below had the duty to behave deferentially and properly to those above, in order to be considered worthy to receive their beneficence. Those who acted in overly direct, rude, or aggressive ways that ran counter to these precepts were often considered bad students.

There are other cross-cultural differences of which to be aware. Some Asian teachers create family-like situations that are strongly based on respect for the teachings and implied social obligations. Teachers may be referred to in Chinese as a surrogate mother or father, while students are called older and younger brothers. A sense of implied responsibilities and obligations pervades all involved. Strong bonding experiences are common, as both students and teachers frequently go out for outings or meals together after class, and those who don't remain outside the inner circle.

Many like this sense of closeness and community. The sense of belonging to a family, tribe, or community has always been and is still a powerful, even primal, human desire. On the negative side this quality sometimes generates confusion and complaints from Western students who, after a while, progressively find the situation becoming weird or frustrating. A student may perceive that knowledge is not being given out based on even-handedness and merit, but instead is denied because the student has transgressed or not met confusing social boundaries that were never clearly spelled out.

Some teachers have a strong conservative Chinese, even Confucian philosophy (rather than a Taoist perspective). Western and Chinese masters alike who have been powerfully influenced by these ancient attitudes may be viscerally attached to them. For example, before the twentieth century, many women were excluded entirely from martial arts instruction in China. Although these attitudes are changing, some Chinese teachers are still less open to teaching women fully.

Another example is the perspective by which, according to Confucian thought, a wise, learned, and experienced teacher passes on superior knowledge to students. These modes of thinking are personified by the classic phrase traditional teachers constantly and repeatedly tell their students in Chinese, "I give you teachings." The Western model is far more the Socratic method, by which students and teachers explore and debate points together.

Although standing up and saying what you think and feel is considered your right these days, if you use this approach towards many traditional Chinese teachers, they could perceive this as insulting, either personally or to the art of tai chi itself. Why? First, it will make the teacher feel as though you didn't trust his authority or knowledge, which is tantamount to calling him a fake. Second, by merely raising a question that the teacher considers inappropriate, he may feel you were deliberately trying to cause him to lose face—an unforgivable act. This may cause him to think of you unkindly and perhaps deliberately withhold information for a short or long period of time. To avoid these situations, it may be a wise idea to learn to sublimate whatever Western models you grew up with and learn to seek out information differently. You can, for example, avoid talking about other teachers' opinions and principles in any way that may be interpreted as challenging your current teacher. Rather than saying so-and-so said this, only talk about the principles involved. State either your own or another's position without mentioning names and ask the teacher's viewpoint about the principle only. Or indirectly quote a dead master's words and ask for an explanation. As the discussion progresses, you can lower yourself slightly by possibly saying, "I thought this was what was meant. Can you tell me how I have misunderstood the issue?" In this way no face is lost and you have shown proper humility. It will have the same effect as a genuine truth-seeking inquiry without transgressing traditional boundaries of face or propriety.

Many Westerners don't appreciate these sophisticated and subtle perspectives. Even more egregious are those students who after they feel they have learned all they can from their teachers, then criticize them behind their backs or go into open conflict with them. This is especially likely to happen if students, accurately or falsely, believe they have exceeded the accomplishments of their teachers and no longer have any use for them. This may cause some Oriental teachers to be less forthcoming with their knowledge to other students downstream, which is sad.

Just as Western students can feel immensely frustrated with traditional Oriental teachers, these same teachers can also have equal frustrations and disappointments with Western students. All systems are open to abuse. It is mostly by being sensitive to the other person's perceptions that cultural misunderstandings between tai chi teachers and students can be kept to a minimum.

Studying Tai Chi in China

Many Westerners arrive in China for short periods either for tourism or business. If you already practice tai chi, you may have charming and unforgettable experiences with Chinese who are flabbergasted that a foreigner does tai chi. And for Westerners, just seeing so many people of all ages doing tai chi can be very inspiring. You might also see a wider variety of regular people, as well as masters, doing a much greater variety of tai chi styles than it is possible to see at home.

The easiest way to see many people doing tai chi, or to find someone to do push hands with, is to go to the public parks in the morning. Your hotel staff may be able to direct you toward the parks that have the most tai chi going on. Higher-level practitioners tend to arrive and leave earlier. By 10.00 a.m., most have gone.

Short two- and three-week tai chi study trips in China are also advertised in tai chi and martial art magazines and these may help you decide whether you want to stay longer.

If you desire more in-depth study trips—several months to years—you will need introductions in order to be accepted by a good teacher. It is important to learn Chinese because you will clearly learn more about tai chi than you would through translators or sign language. Even after learning Chinese, you will still need to understand the country's culture and withstand the feeling of alienation. This is a downside of staying in "exotic" foreign lands, and not everyone is temperamentally suited to living abroad, particularly in China. Many students who begin with a great deal of enthusiasm and idealism about staying a long time "learning with the master" become discouraged and end up leaving the country much earlier than planned.

Conclusion

No matter what age you are, the study of tai chi offers the rich potential to positively affect and inspire many aspects of your life. However, competence in this art is not gained casually. Learning tai chi is challenging for many beginners, much like learning a musical instrument or a sport like golf: practice and heart make it a greater and greater joy. There are always going to be those moments of magic when everything comes together and you feel deeply connected to your soul.

As with any art or sport, the better the teacher, the easier it is to learn and overcome the challenges you will encounter. These will include learning the form's movements and using them to help you release some of the physical, emotional, and intellectual blockages that prevent you from being a fully relaxed, joyful, healthy, and mature human being. The most important thing in tai chi is to find a good teacher and then practice what you have learned.

I wrote this book in the hope that tai chi can become as widely practiced in Western countries as it is in China and other Asian countries. It will help solve health problems people face individually, as well as help mitigate the medical crisis that is being created by the West's aging population. It can gently reduce the stress that is prevalent in so many of us, and at the deepest levels, reverse deeply-rooted spiritual malaise.

What is the Difference Between Tai Chi and Chi Gung?

This is a much more complex question than it seems, and cannot be fully answered in a few simple sentences. There are hundreds of styles of chi gung and five major schools of tai chi with numerous variations. This is a lot of tai chi and a lot of chi gung from which to make a simple statement. Accurately distinguishing between them is like separating out all the color flows and shadings within a single beautiful but complex painting.

There is another issue that muddies the waters and makes answering this question difficult. Many obtain information on the differences and similarities from a local instructor, or from a Chinese instructor who cannot translate from one culture to another easily, or who may not want to share what has been secret, etc. The trouble is that instructors may only know details about the specific type of chi gung they do, and not other types or its relationships to chi-energy arts as a whole. This is not unusual, just as in the field of science, biologists often don't know that much about civil engineering, and vice versa. As a result, misinformation and half-truths abound.

Anything of truly great value always has great subtlety, whether or not it looks simple and easy on the surface. Some other differences not mentioned here are too technical, and will not be covered in this book as they may confuse rather than clarify. To bypass complex technical issues, just as is done when you want common sense to tell you how computers work, we will look at the four most commonly given simple answers to the original question—what is the difference between tai chi and chi gung? Each answer gives a progressively more complete answer. All are only partial truths, but at least they are the most accurate answers that can be given without going into excessive detail.

Level 1: Tai chi is a form of chi gung, or, chi gung is tai chi's parent

This is the most common answer. The accurate part of the statement is this: the invisible chi or internal power aspects included within the tai chi part of tai chi chuan derive directly from one branch of the 3,000-year-old Taoist chi gung tradition, whereas Taoist chi gung does not come from tai chi. However, the statement is misleading because it omits Buddhist or Confucian chi gung, which have little in common with tai chi's roots in Taoist chi gung or Taoism.

This answer also involves a common error in logic: since to the Western ear it sounds as if the word energy is contained in both words, they must mean the same thing. Right? Wrong! The chi of chi gung means energy, the chi of tai chi does not (see pp. 3 and 7). To add to the confusion, the chi in tai chi and chi gung are almost universally pronounced by Westerners as "chee," which is accurate for chi gung and inaccurate for tai chi ("gee") chuan. Those who commonly both see and mispronounce tai chi as chee also tend to assume both mean the same thing, which they do not.

Confusion escalates and gets reinforced when you find out both tai chi and chi gung work with chi-energy (however often in different ways) and have similar benefits. Adding to the potential confusion, although many people may have heard the name, most in the West have only seen tai chi or chi gung in still photos, on television, or at the cinema. When shown visually, if these arts are even named, usually narrators inaccurately call both tai chi, because they don't know the difference. This commonly leaves the impression that chi gung is tai chi or vice versa. The public subsequently has an association that slow-motion movements + Chinese something-or-other = tai chi. Consequently, the public and the media are more familiar with the name tai chi than chi gung, and commonly do not make much distinction between them.

Level 2: Tai chi is a martial art, chi gung is purely for healing

The accurate part of this statement is that chi gung has specific techniques or styles that are particularly effective for specific diseases beyond the ken of tai chi. For instance, there are specific chi gung methods for helping those with cancer and mitigating the effects of radiation and chemotherapy. The misleading part is that although all tai chi powerfully heals and maintains health, only a tiny fraction of participants do any of its practical martial arts techniques. On the other hand, chi gung also has within it practices for increasing the power you need to make self-defense techniques effective, even though chi gung *per se* does not include the fighting techniques themselves.

Level 3: Tai chi and chi gung have different movements

Although the first part of this answer can be a little murky, the second part is relatively clear. Both tai chi and some (but not most or all), aspects of chi gung do what they do using flowing, fluid, slow-motion movements. To an untrained eye, all regular, smooth, slow-motion movements would tend to look the same, no matter how different they are in reality. Yet a casual observer would be able to clearly distinguish between different kinds of movements done at a faster speed. Nevertheless, slow-motion movements are only fast movements done slowly.

The second part of the answer is this: just because tai chi and chi gung movements are done in slow motion does not mean that their movements must basically be the same. There is an exceptionally wide range of different movements, each requiring different kinds of physical coordination. Moreover, although the slow-motion movements of different tai chi styles may be somewhat different, on the whole they are basically variations of the same theme.

In contrast, slow-motion movements in a particular chi gung style can look radically different from either tai chi or other chi gung systems. Take, for example, two well-respected members of the Taoist chi gung tribe—tai chi chuan and Wild Goose chi gung. Wild Goose has as many moves as a tai chi long form, yet looks radically different from tai chi. Likewise, non-Taoist medical and Buddhist chi gung systems also contain movements not to be found in tai chi or each other.

There are many ways to move the body, as can be seen in the differences in the dance world between styles of ballet, ballroom, tap, disco, and hip-hop. Like dance styles, within the hundreds of chi gung schools you can move in other ways besides regular, smooth, slow-motion movements. There are techniques which involve shaking, jumping up and down, vibrating, shouting, alternating speed with staying dead still, flapping like a bird, squatting flatfooted, and even moving freely and spontaneously in ways almost too strange to describe, while making weird, otherworldly sounds.

Above and beyond moving, chi gung also has primary methods that specialize in:

- standing, either with your arms by your sides or in all kinds of positions
- sitting, both on the floor and in chairs
- lying down in various positions
- sexual and all kinds of human interactions.

Although tai chi may use standing, sitting, and lying down techniques, they are ancillary to the primary technique of slow-motion movements for health, longevity, and stress management.

Level 4: Tai chi and chi gung may work with chi-energy differently

Why are you doing these movements in the first place? From a purely physical viewpoint the body needs to move and exercise to prevent problems. A different perspective is that the movements are designed to specifically promote the flow of chi within you. Therefore, if you want to generate a specific chi flow in your body, one type of movement may make it easier whereas others may make it harder.

Tai chi is based upon the potential to fully incorporate all 16 parts of the nei gung system (see p. 226) seamlessly into every movement; chi gung normally tends to partially utilize some, but not all, of the 16 nei gung components in any specific movement or entire form. In tai chi, although some specific moves may make it slightly easier to initially learn or solidly assimilate any one of the 16 components, for an advanced practitioner, the other 15 are ideally always present and integrated within each and every move of the form.

Some Taoist chi gung schools will teach the entire 16 components initially through a series of short chi gung forms, each of which emphasizes two or three specific parts of the nei gung, until the final form which encompasses all 16. After this the student has a complete background within which to engage learning the full energetic potential of tai chi. The author, for example, does this in his teaching work, using six very short chi gung sets, the first five of which initially emphasize only one to three components of the entire 16 nei gung components.

Chi gung also often separates specific chi functions into separate movements or different forms. For example, while doing a chi gung form, during one move you might direct energy through a specific acupuncture meridian (the lung or heart meridian for example), and in the next move you might direct energy through a different meridian. Or in one move, you might draw energy through a particular acupuncture point in your body, and in the next release the energy from a different one. Or within the same form during one series of moves you could deliberately only exclusively activate and work with one of your three tantiens or centers of energy, and later within the same form, in a different series of moves, deliberately solely activate a different tantien and its functions, or other specific elements of the Taoist nei gung system.

Ideally, in tai chi, an experienced practitioner will not separate these energy practices in this way.

The Five Elements

What you do each season of your life matters to your long-term health, as each internal organ and season has its specific needs, and directly affects the subsequent organs and seasons. For example, winter affects your kidneys. During this season it is important to rest the kidneys, the source of your chi and your body vitality in general. Your body is like a harvested field. After the harvest, the field needs rest to ensure that next year's yield is not diminished by the strain of this year's activity. Without the needed rest and regeneration its capacity to provide useable nutrients to seeds and sprouting plants during the spring will be compromised.

Likewise, if the kidneys (water element) are not nourished during the winter, their ability to activate the full potential of the following spring season's liver's chi (wood element) for the next yearly cycle will be weakened. To weaken one element during its natural season is to weaken the element of the next season.

Conversely, if you strengthen the previous season's organ (the kidneys, for example), not only will you feel better during the next season, but that season's organ (the liver) will have the opportunity to reach its full potential for the coming year.

If the soil's vitality is insufficient, the new spring seeds may lack enough support to release their power fully. Equally, if the seeds do not get enough water, sunlight, or whatever during the spring season, the new plants are less likely to grow fully during the summer season. In the same way, whether the liver is or isn't well cared for in the spring will determine if your heart will or won't do well during the summer season.

Metal

The lungs and large intestine are associated with the element of metal and the harvest of autumn.

Physical Effects

The lungs extract chi from the air. They are central to breathing and obtaining oxygen, which are absolutely vital for all metabolic functions. Lungs create a protective layer of energy (called *wei chi* in Chinese) between the skin and the muscles, which enables us to resist infections. The lungs dominate all skin functions, making your body's skin beautiful and smooth. If the lungs are compromised, your skin lacks luster and shows signs of aging or disease.

Emotional Effects

The lungs are associated with the positive emotions of enthusiasm and willingness to engage with life. Conversely, they are also associated with the negative emotions of grief—excessive dwelling on the past and the inability to let go of sadness.

Seasonal Effects

Autumn is the season when your body reaps the benefits, or weaknesses, of how it has been treated during the previous year. Strong lungs make you less prone to the colds that more frigid weather brings. The consequence of not building the lungs up during autumn is that it compromises the following season's kidney functions. This results in general kidney problems such as a lack of vitality, not being able to rest or sleep properly, and sexual weakness or dissatisfaction. Chinese medicine says, "lungs descend the chi and the kidneys grab it." If the lung–kidney connection is poor you can become prone both to bouts of asthma and urinary problems.

Water

The kidneys and bladder are associated with the water element and winter.

Physical Effects

Healthy kidneys kick-start the generation and circulation of the energy that moves through all your other internal organs. Without this kick-start your other internal organs never get into full gear. The kidneys are responsible for general vitality, sexuality, childhood development, and the strength of bones.

The kidneys also preserve and nourish the original genetic chi and constitutional strength your parents gave you. They are responsible, along with the liver, for correct blood pressure, and for sperm and ova being healthy. The kidneys help hair to maintain its luster, and keep its bright natural color without turning gray before its time.

Unhealthy kidneys sap your general vitality, cause you to gain weight, and severely weaken your body's energetic inheritance. The kidneys can be weakened through a workaholic or excessive partying lifestyle, drug abuse, or sexual addiction beyond the constitutional strength of your body to handle. These can burn your kidneys out like a Roman Candle or lead to chronic fatigue syndrome.

Fertility rates are declining throughout the Western world. It also can be observed that many people under the age of 35 show the diminished vitality and functional age of people significantly older. These conditions may be the result of kidney weakness. Kidney imbalances also cause kidney infections, kidney stones, urinary tract infections, incontinence, sexual problems (impotence and frigidity), and fluid retention.

Emotional Effects

The kidneys are associated with such positive emotions as being willing and able to patiently engage in life fully, with courage, and without easily getting bored. Strong kidneys also produce "a will that can't be willed"—an effortless willpower that is the natural consequence of a strong life force.

The kidneys are also associated with negative emotions of fear. Weak kidneys often result in light or medium bouts of depression where you feel sad and lethargic, rather than catatonic. Boosting the kidneys can help severe or clinical depression, but cannot usually completely cure the condition. Weak kidneys can also create pushiness that is reflexive rather than deliberate, and an unhealthy over-willfulness.

Seasonal Effects

The consequence of not resting the kidneys fully during the winter (for example through excessive work or not sleeping enough) is the diminished capacity of the liver in the following spring. This compromises your ability to start and follow through all aspects of your life—work, family, and play—during the next year. You are de-energized and never get going properly when your liver is sluggish rather than full of vigor.

Wood

The liver and gallbladder are associated with the wood element and spring.

Physical Effects

A healthy liver allows the smooth flow of chi and fluids throughout the body, which in turn creates physical strength and stamina. The liver is responsible for the strength and flexibility of your muscles, tendons, and ligaments. In terms of functional strength and power, these tendons and ligaments are as important, if not more so, than muscles. Ligaments, not the muscles as is commonly believed, hold up, support, and prevent your body from collapsing under gravity.

Chi usually stagnates in the liver, causing other kinds of chi to stagnate downstream according to the flow of the five elements. The liver is also related to such gynecological issues as irregular menstruation, excessive bleeding, PMS, and breast tenderness. When the chi of the liver does not flow smoothly, it often results in repressed anger that leads to depression, a compressed, imploded body, and high blood pressure.

Emotional Effects

The liver is associated with the positive emotions of perseverance and confidence. The liver is the source of your ability to overcome obstacles and to deal effectively with life's ever-present frustrations. According to Chinese medicine, the liver is the planner. So if your initial plan gets blocked, you can either push through or go to plan B. Your natural ability to adjust gets compromised if the liver chi is stagnant. Within the liver lies what is known in Chinese as the *hun*, the psychic or intuitive part of our spirit or soul. It empowers us to recognize our higher purpose in life—our life plan.

The liver is associated with the negative emotions of excessive anger and irritability. Suppressing anger is often linked with depression, as are the functions and chi of the liver and kidneys. At a less severe level, a diminished liver is responsible for the depression of PMS, which finishes when menstruation is over. An extremely deficient liver is directly tied to severe and clinical depression.

Seasonal Effects

The consequence of not building the liver up in the spring is the compromising of the fire element of your heart and blood circulation in the summer. This is because chi (the smooth flow of which is governed by the liver) moves your blood. This is especially important for men, who are more prone than women toward heart and circulatory conditions and testosterone-generated anger. This scorches rather than nourishes plants during the prime-growing season.

Fire

The heart and the small intestine are associated with the fire element and summer.

Physical Effects

The heart pumps your blood and maintains good circulation. It is responsible for the shine, color, and health of your facial complexion.

A weak heart can lead to such heart conditions as palpitations, angina, and full-blown heart attacks. From the Western, but not the Chinese, perspective a strong heart function can improve excessively high or low blood pressure

Emotional Effects

The heart is associated with the positive emotions of love, joy, and happiness. The heart is the body's center of consciousness. It is responsible for the clarity of your mental functions. It generates the spirit referred to in Chinese medicine, described on p. 22 (this is not the same as religious spirituality—see p. 190), which can be seen in the shine behind the eyes showing intelligence and awareness. According to Chinese medicine, the heart also keeps the spirit, which enables the mind to be settled and calm.

The heart is also associated with the negative emotions of sorrow, sadness, hysteria, and morbidity. It is responsible for mentally destabilizing people, who often end up incessantly talking to themselves, a condition the Chinese poetically call "phlegm misting the heart." When the spirit or consciousness that resides in the heart is disturbed you experience anxiety, panic attacks, insomnia, and an inability to think clearly.

Seasonal Effects

Not building up the heart during the summer can result in the spleen being compromised.

Earth

The spleen and stomach are associated with the earth element and the period of Indian summer.

Physical Effects

A healthy spleen enables you to extract, build energy, and obtain vibrant vitality from the everyday activities that nourish us, such as eating, drinking, breathing, and exercising. The spleen also dominates or controls the functions of the muscles. It holds up and keeps the internal organs in their proper places and alignments. The spleen provides the force that keeps the blood in the blood vessels.

An unhealthy spleen may cause the internal organs to fall out of alignment, resulting in a prolapsed uterus or bowels. Through the weakening of the binding force between blood and blood vessels, various problems can occur such as varicose veins, bruising under the skin, uterine bleeding or spotting, and red spots under the skin. Deficient chi of the spleen can also cause candida, a build up of yeast. Candida can lower energy, fog thinking, and cause weight gain, depression, constipation, diarrhea, gas, and bloating. Although it can be transmitted to men sexually, yeast infections are more prevalent in women.

A weak or damaged spleen makes it easy for a person to lack focus, become disassociated, physically devitalized, and spaced out. Your mind feels heavy and lethargic, as though you have cotton wool in your head.

Emotional Effects
The spleen is associated with emotional stability and being grounded, mental focus, and concentration. It also enables you to absorb and assimilate information from your environment, either from natural observation, intuition, or learned behavior.

Negative aspects include indecisiveness, worry, anxiety, melancholy, and obsessive behavior.

Seasonal Effects
The consequence of a weakened earth element for the following autumn season is that you are deprived of the necessary inner stability to energetically launch the next complete yearly cycle well. The cycle begins with the lungs. The relevant phrase is that the spleen creates phlegm while the lungs hold it. As the colder autumn and winter seasons arrive you become prone to the problems of phlegm and weakened lungs. These include a runny nose, stuffiness, colds, pneumonia, bronchitis, flu, and excess mucus.

The Five Elements and Tai Chi
The practices for adjusting the internal components of your tai chi form as the energetic flow shifts from season to season are a fundamental part of Taoist tai chi. Understanding how the five elements work is also a higher level aspect of secular tai chi. The principles of the five elements can be incorporated in the movements of any tai chi form, both for promoting health and for self-defense. Taoist tai chi and secular tai chi are described in detail in Chapter 8.

How Does Tai Chi Differ from Yoga?

Health and longevity are primary goals of both tai chi and hatha yoga, and many people cross-train in both disciplines. Some of the means both use to achieve these ends are similar, but others are quite different. Both consider stretching to be equally beneficial for health and healing, and use it extensively, although often in different ways.

Here is a very simple way to explain the difference: in tai chi, you relax to stretch; in yoga, you stretch to relax.

Similarities

Tai chi and yoga are reliable systems that have stood the test of time and have clearly emerged into the mainstream as beneficial health exercises. Both emphasize the mind's partnership and primacy over the physical, so awareness becomes the door into the deeper, more subtle possibilities of the body. Both emphasize stretching, body alignments, breath work, and chi-energy, called prana in yoga. Both seek to integrate the body, subtle energy, and mind. Their approaches to physicality are significantly more subtle than ordinary Western exercise methods and sports. Both help you calm your mind and deal with stress.

Differences

Many different variations of yoga have developed and are continuing to evolve in the West. I studied traditional hatha yoga during my high school and college years. This was followed by two years of training in India which included extensive pranayama work. My conclusions about the differences between tai chi and yoga are based on these experiences.

From a technical perspective, yoga and tai chi emphasize different points, as the following examples will show.

TAI CHI'S EMPHASIS	YOGA'S EMPHASIS
Advocates never holding the breath.	Yoga has practices to hold the breath for short or extended periods of time.
Tai chi does not breathe into the front of the chest, rather it sinks and drops the chest, and does not thrust it forward (as in a military posture).	Its normal posture uses the front of the chest to breathe, pushing it forward and raising it, albeit more gently than is done in a military posture.
Advocates relaxing the chest.	Advocates relaxing the chest when not holding the breath.
Stretch and benefits through sophisticated flowing movements.	Stretch and benefits through holding postures rather than moving.
You get the muscles to stretch by getting the ligaments to release, using fluid motion.	You hold the position and try to make the muscles go further. The emphasis is on getting the long muscles of the body to stretch.
Postures are always done continuously moving with one or both feet on the floor.	Postures are done standing, sitting, or lying on the floor, or inverted with the feet facing upwards (shoulder and head stands).
The legs are always at least slightly bent and can go as far as being in a low squat.	
A straight spine in tai chi is erect, not arched, with a small rather than a large S-curve.	Postures normally arch the back.
In virtually all moves, the spine does not bend forwards, backwards, or sideways.	Some postures dramatically extend the spine sideways, forwards, or backwards (as in touching the toes or back bends).
The head and neck do not fully bend sideways or forwards, and should never bend backwards at all.	Full head and neck bends forwards, backwards, and sideways are common.
The joints are never fully bent, straightened, or locked.	Many postures fully bend, straighten, or lock the joints.
In general, uses less extreme degrees of stretching that are more like normal body movements.	Includes extreme stretches, such as full splits or crossing both feet behind the head.
Requires and emphasizes developing physical coordination and movement skills.	Emphasis not placed on developing coordination and movement skills.

TAI CHI'S EMPHASIS	YOGA'S EMPHASIS
Flow and let go.	Control.
Each posture works all the joints, internal organs, and spine simultaneously.	Uses distinctly separate postures to work on specific joints or organs at a time.
More circular approach. Every movement should be externally and internally circular.	More linear approach, although some schools may include some circular elements.
Energetics based on the 16-part Taoist nei gung system (see p.226) and the principles of traditional Chinese medicine.	Energetics based on pranayama, kundalini, the chakra system, and the principles of Ayurveda.

Tai chi is a fully developed martial art. Yoga is not. Here is a wonderful story that illustrates this difference.

Cheng Man Ching, an elderly tai chi chuan master, lived and taught in New York City during the 1960s and 1970s. He was also familiar with high-level yoga. Once he was asked about the essential difference between tai chi and yoga. After due consideration he said that both could help you understand the mysteries of chi, explore the possibilities of spiritual potential, and become healthy and strong.

Then, with a wry smile, he said the difference would arise if both a yogi, who was flexible enough to put his leg behind his head, and a tai chi chuan practitioner were sitting and meditating when a violent and determined person attacked. He mused that the yogi, who was flexible enough to put his leg behind his head, and strong enough to stand on his hands would get knocked off his meditation pillow, while the tai chi adept would not. Remaining seated, he would physically deal with the attacker, and would peacefully continue meditating.

There is some crossover between both disciplines from the perspective of dynamic movements versus static postures. While standing only, rather than sitting or lying down, tai chi does hold static single postures, although with the goal of producing body strength and internal co-ordination rather than stretch and flexibility, as in yoga. Equally, some yoga systems such as Pattabhi Jois's Ashtanga Yoga, weave yoga postures into short sets of movements, albeit with much fewer and less sophisticated movements than tai chi uses.

If you do practice both yoga and tai chi, which practice you do first depends upon the following:

- if you do a very soft form of yoga that strongly emphasizes deep relaxation to enter into a stretch, it will not matter if you do yoga or tai chi first
- if, however, you do a form of yoga that emphasizes power development, tensing first in order to achieve a stretch afterward, or practicing in extreme heat, either do yoga before tai chi, or do each separately at different times of the day.

Further Information

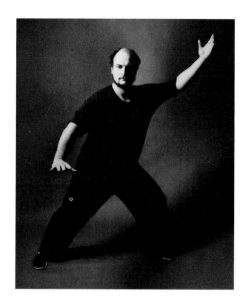

Bruce Frantzis is the founder of Energy Arts, Inc., based in Northern California. Energy Arts offers instructor certification programs, retreats, and corporate and public seminars in North America and Europe. Frantzis teaches Energy Arts courses in tai chi, chi gung, meditation, Longevity Breathing®, hsing-i, ba gua, and related subjects.

For the latest details of events, instructional materials, and certified instructors, visit the Energy Arts website, www.energyarts.com

Books by Bruce Frantzis

Opening the Energy Gates of Your Body

The Power of Internal Martial Arts

The Water Method of Taoist Meditation, Volume 1: Relaxing Into Your Being

The Water Method of Taoist Meditation, Volume 2: The Great Stillness

DVDs/Videos

Longevity Breathing

Taoist Energy Arts

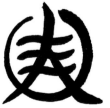

Energy Arts, Inc.,
P. O. Box 99, Fairfax,
CA 94978-0099, USA
Phone: (415) 454-5243
Fax: (415) 454-0907
www.energyarts.com

Index

Make
www.thorsonselement.com
your online sanctuary

Get online information, inspiration and guidance to help you on the path to physical and spiritual well-being. Drawing on the integrity and vision of our authors and titles, and with health advice, articles, astrology, tarot, a meditation zone, author interviews and events listings, www.thorsonselement.com is a great alternative to help create space and peace in our lives.

So if you've always wondered about practising yoga, following an allergy-free diet, using the tarot or getting a life coach, we can point you in the right direction.

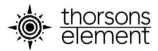

thorsons
element